T0263256

Sexually Transmitted Infections

Editor

COURTNEY J. PITTS

NURSING CLINICS
OF NORTH AMERICA

www.nursing.theclinics.com

Consulting Editor
STEPHEN D. KRAU

September 2020 • Volume 55 • Number 3

ELSEVIER

1600 John F. Kennedy Boulevard • Suite 1800 • Philadelphia, Pennsylvania, 19103-2899

http://www.theclinics.com

NURSING CLINICS OF NORTH AMERICA Volume 55, Number 3
September 2020 ISSN 0029-6465, ISBN-13: 978-0-323-75454-5

Editor: Kerry Holland
Developmental Editor: Casey Potter

© **2020 Elsevier Inc. All rights reserved.**

This periodical and the individual contributions contained in it are protected under copyright by Elsevier, and the following terms and conditions apply to their use:

Photocopying
Single photocopies of single articles may be made for personal use as allowed by national copyright laws. Permission of the Publisher and payment of a fee is required for all other photocopying, including multiple or systematic copying, copying for advertising or promotional purposes, resale, and all forms of document delivery. Special rates are available for educational institutions that wish to make photocopies for non-profit educational classroom use. For information on how to seek permission visit www.elsevier.com/permissions or call: (+44) 1865 843830 (UK)/ (+1) 215 239 3804 (USA).

Derivative Works
Subscribers may reproduce tables of contents or prepare lists of articles including abstracts for internal circulation within their institutions. Permission of the Publisher is required for resale or distribution outside the institution. Permission of the Publisher is required for all other derivative works, including compilations and translations (please consult www.elsevier.com/permissions).

Electronic Storage or Usage
Permission of the Publisher is required to store or use electronically any material contained in this periodical, including any article or part of an article (please consult www.elsevier.com/permissions). Except as outlined above, no part of this publication may be reproduced, stored in a retrieval system or transmitted in any form or by any means, electronic, mechanical, photocopying, recording or otherwise, without prior written permission of the Publisher.

Notice
No responsibility is assumed by the Publisher for any injury and/or damage to persons or property as a matter of products liability, negligence or otherwise, or from any use or operation of any methods, products, instructions or ideas contained in the material herein. Because of rapid advances in the medical sciences, in particular, independent verification of diagnoses and drug dosages should be made.

Although all advertising material is expected to conform to ethical (medical) standards, inclusion in this publication does not constitute a guarantee or endorsement of the quality or value of such product or of the claims made of it by its manufacturer.

Nursing Clinics of North America (ISSN 0029-6465) is published quarterly by Elsevier Inc., 360 Park Avenue South, New York, NY 10010-1710. Months of issue are March, June, September, and December. Periodicals postage paid at New York, NY and additional mailing offices. Subscription price per year is, $163.00 (US individuals), $518.00 (US institutions), $275.00 (international individuals), $631.00 (international institutions), $231.00 (Canadian individuals), $631.00 (Canadian institutions), $100.00 (US and Canadian students), and $135.00 (international students). To receive student/resident rate, orders must be accompanied by name of affiliated institution, date of term, and the signature of program/residency coordinator on institution letterhead. Orders will be billed at individual rate until proof of status is received. Foreign air speed delivery is included in all *Clinics* subscription prices. All prices are subject to change without notice. **POSTMASTER:** Send address changes to *Nursing Clinics*, Elsevier Health Sciences Division, Subscription Customer Service, 3251 Riverport Lane, Maryland Heights, MO 63043. **Customer Service: Telephone: 1-800-654-2452** (U.S. and Canada); **1-314-447-8871 (outside U.S. and Canada). Fax: 1-314-447-8029. E-mail: journalscustomerservice-usa@ elsevier.com** (for print support) and **journalsonlinesupport-usa@elsevier.com** (for online support).

Nursing Clinics of North America is covered in *EMBASE/Excerpta Medica, MEDLINE/PubMed (Index Medicus), Social Sciences Citation Index, Current Contents, ASCA, Cumulative Index to Nursing, RNdex Top 100,* and Allied Health Literature and International Nursing Index (INI).

Contributors

CONSULTING EDITOR

STEPHEN D. KRAU, PhD, RN, CNE
Associate Professor (Ret), Vanderbilt University School of Nursing, Nashville, Tennessee

EDITOR

COURTNEY J. PITTS, DNP, MPH, FNP-BC
Associate Professor, FNP Program Director, Vanderbilt University School of Nursing, Nashville, Tennessee

AUTHORS

ANGELINA ANTHAMATTEN, DNP, FNP-BC
Assistant Professor, Vanderbilt University School of Nursing, Nashville, Tennessee

CINDY BROHOLM, MS, MPH, FNP-BC
Assistant Professor of Nursing, Harriet Rothkopf Heilbrunn School of Nursing, Long Island University, Brooklyn, New York

HOLLY CLINE, MSN, ANP-C
Vanderbilt University School of Nursing, Nashville, Tennessee

SHAMEKA L. CODY, PhD, AGNP-C
Assistant Professor, Capstone College of Nursing, The University of Alabama, Tuscaloosa, Alabama

SHANNON COLE, DNP, APRN-BC
Assistant Professor of Nursing, Vanderbilt University School of Nursing, Nashville, Tennessee

MELISSA DAVIS, DNP, CNM, FNP
Assistant Professor, Vanderbilt University School of Nursing, Nashville, Tennessee

NICOLE DELLISE, DNP, FNP-BC
Instructor, Vanderbilt University School of Nursing, Nashville, Tennessee

TRAVIS DUNLAP, PhD, ANP-C
Vanderbilt University School of Nursing, Nashville, Tennessee

MELISSA GLASSFORD, DNP, FNP
Assistant Professor, Vanderbilt University School of Nursing, Nashville, Tennessee

QUEEN HENRY-OKAFOR, PhD, FNP-BC, PMHNP-BC
Assistant Professor, Vanderbilt University School of Nursing, Nashville, Tennessee

LESLIE HOPKINS, DNP, FNP-C, ANP-C
Vanderbilt University School of Nursing, Nashville, Tennessee

TAMIKA HUDSON, DNP, APRN, FNP-C
Assistant Professor of Nursing, Vanderbilt University School of Nursing, Nashville, Tennessee

ALLYSON KORNAHRENS, DNP, RN, FNP-C, ENP-C, CNL, CRN, CCRN
Clinical Instructor, Director of the Advanced Practice Nursing Program in Family Health, Department of Graduate Studies: Family Health, Stony Brook University School of Nursing, Stony Brook, New York

ROBIN M. LAWSON, DNP, CRNP, ACNP-BC, NP-C, FAANP
Clinical Professor, Capstone College of Nursing, The University of Alabama, Tuscaloosa, Alabama

AMY S.D. LEE, DNP, ARNP, WHNP-BC
Clinical Associate Professor, Capstone College of Nursing, The University of Alabama, Tuscaloosa, Alabama

MARY LAUREN PFIEFFER, DNP, FNP-BC, CPN
Assistant Professor, Vanderbilt University School of Nursing, Nashville, Tennessee

MARY MCNAMARA, DNP, FNP-BC
Clinical Assistant Professor, Department of Population Health Nursing Science, University of Illinois at Chicago College of Nursing, Chicago, Illinois

COURTNEY J. PITTS, DNP, MPH, FNP-BC
Associate Professor, FNP Program Director, Vanderbilt University School of Nursing, Nashville, Tennessee

ANNA RICHMOND, DNP, FNP-C, PNP-PC
Assistant Professor, Vanderbilt University School of Nursing, Nashville, Tennessee

SHELZA RIVAS, DNP, WHNP, AGPCNP
Instructor of Nursing, Vanderbilt University School of Nursing, Nashville, Tennessee

JULIA M. STEED, PhD, APRN, FNP-BC
Assistant Professor, Vanderbilt University School of Nursing, Nashville, Tennessee

SHIRLEY STEPHENSON, MS, MFA, MA, FNP-BC
Teaching Associate, Department of Population Health Nursing Science, University of Illinois at Chicago College of Nursing, Chicago, Illinois

JANNYSE TAPP, DNP, FNP-BC
Assistant Professor of Nursing, Vanderbilt University School of Nursing, Nashville, Tennessee

JUSTIN M. WARYOLD, DNP, RN, ANP-C, ACNP-BC, GS-C, CNE, FAANP
Clinical Assistant Professor, Director of the Advanced Practice Nursing Program in Adult Health, Department of Graduate Studies: Adult Health, Clinical Instructor, Department of Medicine, Stony Brook University School of Medicine, Stony Brook, New York

CHARLES YINGLING, DNP, FNP-BC, FAANP
Clinical Assistant Professor, Associate Dean for Practice and Community Partnerships, Department of Population Health Nursing Science, University of Illinois at Chicago College of Nursing, Chicago, Illinois

Contents

Rates of sexually transmitted infections (STI) are on the rise in the United States. Some STIs are at an all-time high. Research has shown that there is a higher prevalence of STIs among some racial and ethnic groups as compared with whites. Factors contributing to this endemic have been explored. Although some individual-level risk factors have previously been identified, data overwhelmingly suggest that social determinants of health are key factors in the overall increase in STIs. Additionally, these social factors have contributed to disparities in STI acquisition. Population-specific interventions targeting social factors are necessary in reducing the rates of STIs.

Evidence-based guidelines have improved diagnosis and treatment of sexually transmitted infections (STI). Social stigma remains a barrier to STI testing and is associated with underutilization of prevention services. Alternatives for STI testing (eg, in-home testing) are convenient. However, some individuals decline follow-up treatment in fear of unintentional disclosure of their diagnosis. This article reviews STI treatment guidelines and examines the impact of stigma and ethical issues on testing, adherence, partner notification, and transmission rates. An understanding of STI-associated ethical issues and controversies is an important step toward eliminating stigma and reducing STI prevalence and morbidity.

Sexually transmitted infections (STIs) are a prevalent global health care problem. Incidence rates are rising yearly. STI incidence is highest for adolescents and young adults ages 15 to 24, who are diagnosed with half of all new STIs. *Chlamydia trachomatis* and *Neisseria gonorrhea* are common STIs caused by bacteria. Treatment guidelines change frequently as a result of antimicrobial resistance and public health trends. It is important for primary care providers to remain up to date with new guidelines. This article provides updates on pharmacologic treatment as well as patient education and follow-up specific to the primary care setting.

Sexually transmitted infections (STIs) are diseases that are transmitted from one person to another person through acts of vaginal, anal, or oral intercourse. The increased presence of STIs among men who have sex with men (MSM) results in a higher rate of STI-related diagnoses, such as proctitis. Proctitis is a common, but often misdiagnosed condition experienced by MSM who present to primary care, urgent care, and emergency settings. It is important that health care providers be knowledgeable of the pathophysiology, risk factors, and clinical presentation of proctitis among MSM for accurate and timely management.

Genital herpes simplex virus infections are among the most prevalent sexually transmitted infections in the United States. It continues to be a public health concern because of its recurrent nature and potential for complications. Treatment is not curative, but rather serves to shorten the duration of symptoms and improve quality of life. Current therapies include episodic treatment and chronic suppressive therapy and are generally well tolerated and effective.

Hepatitis C virus (HCV) is a common infectious disease affecting people worldwide. In the past 10 years, the incidence of HCV has steadily increased in the United States. With the advent of new direct-acting antiviral medications, the treatment of HCV has become important and can cure the infection.

Despite the near-eradication of syphilis in the United States in the late 1990s, new infections have surged over the past 20 years. Dubbed, "the great imitator," syphilis infections often can be misdiagnosed and resultantly untreated. This leads to people inadvertently infecting others. This article reviews the history of syphilis, including the unethical studies undertaken in the past; current epidemiology; treatment guidelines; and strategies to reduce new infections.

Several evidence-based resources are available to assist clinicians in screening, diagnosis, and management of sexually transmitted infections.

Mobile medical technology can make accessing quality clinical information more efficient for health care professionals. This review focuses on medical information on the Internet and mobile medical applications that provide valuable clinical information for health care professionals caring for individuals with sexually transmitted infections. Appraisal of the quality of medical information on the Internet and mobile applications is also discussed.

There is a need to increase improve the delivery of health care for sexual minorities. The lesbian, gay, bisexual, transgender, and queer (LGBTQ) community has historically experienced bias, discrimination, and perceived inadequate or inappropriate care. Reduction of this barrier can begin by providers addressing implicit bias and creating a welcoming, safe environment for all persons seeking care. Using preferred name and pronouns and obtaining a sexual health history that is individualized and free from assumption is imperative. This article provides interventions to diminish barriers to care and foster provider preparedness for the care of LGBTQ individuals.

This article provides an overview of the incidence and prevalence of sexually transmitted infections in pregnant women in the United States. It discusses screening guidelines and best practices related to treatments. Safety, pharmacology, and monitoring of both the woman and her fetus are detailed.

It has been more than 38 years since the first reported case of human immunodeficiency virus (HIV). Over this period of time, there has been an evolution in the care, management, and survival of those living with HIV and acquired immunodeficiency syndrome (AIDS). Current efforts to stabilize HIV incidence have targeted pharmacologic management with antiretroviral therapy (ART) coupled with programs that focus on individual characteristics, social norms, and structural barriers. It is important that clinicians are knowledgeable of prevention efforts and up-to-date clinical practice guidelines in order to best provide care for people living with HIV.

This article reviews the disparities in human immunodeficiency virus (HIV) incidence, presents evidence on the efficacy of preexposure prophylaxis (PrEP) and nonoccupational postexposure prophylaxis (nPEP), provides an overview of clinical guidelines for prescribing PrEP and nPEP, discusses strategies to promote efficient use of these effective interventions, and reviews best practices in treatment retention for people at high risk for HIV. Nurses are optimally positioned to prevent new HIV infections. When working with sensitive topics such as sexual practices and substance use, nurses excel at building rapport, making shared decisions, and educating about risk reduction with an affirming, nonjudgmental approach.

Robin M. Lawson

The human immunodeficiency virus (HIV) and sexually transmitted infections (STIs) are considered epidemics in the United States. Research on the association between STIs and HIV infectiousness and susceptibility has shown that STIs promote HIV acquisition and transmission via mucosal inflammation and ulceration caused by viral or bacterial pathogens. Some of the most common STIs associated with HIV are chlamydia, gonorrhea, syphilis, and herpes simplex virus type 2. STIs are a major cause of morbidity and mortality, particularly if diagnosis or treatment is delayed. Prevention and treatment of both HIV and STIs is essential to ending these associated epidemics.

NURSING CLINICS OF NORTH AMERICA

SERIES OF RELATED INTEREST

Critical Care Nursing Clinics of North America
https://www.ccnursing.theclinics.com/
Advances in Family Practice Nursing
http://www.advancesinfamilypracticenursing.com/

THE CLINICS ARE AVAILABLE ONLINE!
Access your subscription at:
www.theclinics.com

Foreword

Sexually Transmitted Diseases in the Midst of the Coronavirus Pandemic

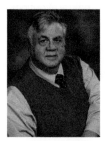

Stephen D. Krau, PhD, RN, CNE
Consulting Editor

The inception of this issue of *Nursing Clinics of North America* occurred prior to the Coronavirus Pandemic, which has taken center stage of the universal health care system. The impact of the pandemic on sexual activity has not been a primary focus, but there is evidence that there has been a change in sexual activity.[1]

The purpose of one study, currently in press, was to explore changes in people's sexual behavior and to "explore the context in which they exist."[1] A convenience sample was given to 270 men and 189 women, who completed a survey related to sexual activities during the pandemic. All subjects were living in Han, China and were Chinese.

While there was a wide range of variation in the results, the study identified that 44% of the participants reported a decrease in the number of sexual partners, while 37% reported a decrease in sexual frequency.[1] In addition, results indicated that those persons who had previously engaged in higher-risk sexual behaviors had a rapid decline in those behaviors. The study indicated that 25% of the participants experienced a decrease in sexual desire, while 18% of men and 8% of women experienced an increase in sexual desire.

To date, this is the only study related to coronavirus and sexual activity and sexual desire. The imitations of the study are obvious with a small sample, self-report data, and lack of generalizability on many levels, including geographical limitations. As we focus on the COVID-19 crisis, it seems other infectious diseases, unless they are underlying issues for COVID patients, are not a central focus.

With the mitigation protocol of "social distancing," the implications for contagion of many infectious diseases would seem likely. It will be of interest in the future to compile data on the prevalence and incidence of new sexually transmitted diseases worldwide when the coronavirus pandemic is under better control. It will also be important to

Nurs Clin N Am 55 (2020) xi–xii
https://doi.org/10.1016/j.cnur.2020.06.010
0029-6465/20/© 2020 Published by Elsevier Inc.

nursing.theclinics.com

know to what extent, if any, sexually transmitted diseases contributed to longer hospital stays and mortality among COVID-19 patients, as well as patients with nonsexually transmitted diseases.

Stephen D. Krau, PhD, RN, CNE
Vanderbilt University School of Nursing
6809 Highland Park Drive
Nashville, TN 37205, USA

E-mail address:
sdkrau@outlook.com

REFERENCE

1. Li W, Li G, Xin C, et al. Changes in sexual behaviors of young women and men during the coronavirus disease 2019 outbreak: a convenience sample from the epidemic area. J Sex Med, in press.

Preface

Sexually Transmitted Infections: Overlooked, Underestimated, and Undiagnosed

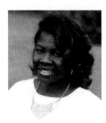

Courtney J. Pitts, DNP, MPH, FNP-BC
Editor

For centuries, health care professionals have diligently worked to manage the health and lives of those they serve in an effort to reduce morbidity and mortality from various diseases. The evolution of evidence-based practices, health policies, and prevention programs has shifted disease management from tertiary preventive methods to more primary preventive methods. Morbidity and mortality, particularly in more developed countries, were historically tied to more infectious disease processes. With the implementation of public health interventions, there was a transition from infectious disease processes to chronic disease processes as the leading causes of death or disease-related complications. Unfortunately, the past decade has seen a slow shift back to infectious disease processes playing a leading role in the deterioration of health among the human population.

An example of infectious disease processes related to significant morbidity and some mortality is sexually transmitted infections (STIs). To date, there is an ongoing epidemic related to STIs that is disproportionately affecting subpopulations within the United States. The identification of antibiotics to treat some STIs has proven beneficial. Appropriate and timely treatment reduces the likelihood of negative health outcomes experienced by women, men, and children alike. In addition, surveillance data from organizations such as the Centers for Disease Control and Prevention have resulted in the identification of new risk factors for the acquisition of STIs. These risk factors provide hints to those most affected: adolescents/young adults and gay or bisexual men. These 2 groups have the highest rates of new infections, but are also the most vulnerable as it pertains to STI acquisition. Addressing subpopulations in a way that is culturally appropriate for that population reduces the likelihood

Nurs Clin N Am 55 (2020) xiii–xiv
https://doi.org/10.1016/j.cnur.2020.06.011
0029-6465/20/© 2020 Published by Elsevier Inc.

of undiagnosed cases that could lead to increased transmission rates among these groups.

The purpose of this issue of *Nursing Clinics of North America* is to provide health care providers with current information related to the prevalence and incidence of STIs. This issue addresses STI clinical presentation, impact on subpopulations, and guidelines related to management across the lifespan. It highlights the psychosocial and ethical aspects of care that should be considered when screening and managing STIs. It includes an article that addresses the relationship between STIs and social determinants of health as vulnerability and access to care commonly result in a lack of diagnosis as well as negative short- and long-term health outcomes. The importance of prevention of STIs is stressed throughout this issue as there are significant implications for mortality with some STIs, such as human immunodeficiency virus. Last, this issue provides health care providers with technological resources that ease the process of screening and management of STIs in a more efficient manner. It is my hope that this issue provides the reader with new knowledge to assist in the preventive and treatment efforts of STIs to help reverse the effects of an epidemic that is overlooked, underestimated, and often undiagnosed.

Courtney J. Pitts, DNP, MPH, FNP-BC
Vanderbilt University School of Nursing
461 21st Avenue South, 352 Frist Hall
Nashville, TN 37240, USA

E-mail address:
courtney.j.pitts@vanderbilt.edu

Sexually Transmitted Infections Prevalence in the United States and the Relationship to Social Determinants of Health

Jannyse Tapp, DNP, FNP-BC*, Tamika Hudson, DNP, APRN, FNP-C

KEYWORDS

- Sexually transmitted infections • Social determinants of health • Poverty • Race
- Income • Disparities

KEY POINTS

- The incidence and prevalence of sexually transmitted infections is increasing in the United States.
- Social determinants of health impact the acquisition of STIs.
- Interventions to decrease the growing rates of STIs should be tailored to the population and associated social determinants.

It has long been recognized that social factors impact health and health status. These factors, the social determinants of health (SDH), have been widely studied and have become the basis of a large body of evidence that reveals the direct connection society plays on shaping health. According to the World Health Organization (WHO), the SDH "are the conditions in which people are born, grow, live, work and age. These circumstances are shaped by the distribution of money, power and resources at global, national and local levels."[1] WHO suggests that health inequities are a direct result of the SDH.[1] Contrary to what some may believe, although medical care directly affects health, evidence has shown that it is not the sole influence on health.[2] Social determinants, such as income, education, and occupation, have direct associations with health indicators and disparities.[2]

Sexually transmitted infections (STI), often used interchangeably in the literature with sexually transmitted diseases, are among the many health conditions that are directly and indirectly impacted by various social determinants.[3] Research has shown

Vanderbilt University School of Nursing, 461 21st Avenue South, Nashville, TN 37240, USA
* Corresponding author.
E-mail address: Jannyse.Tapp@vanderbilt.edu

Nurs Clin N Am 55 (2020) 283–293
https://doi.org/10.1016/j.cnur.2020.05.001
0029-6465/20/© 2020 Elsevier Inc. All rights reserved.

nursing.theclinics.com

that there is a higher prevalence of STIs among some racial and ethnic groups as compared with whites.[4] However, it is important to know that these disparities do not exist because of the ethnic differences, but rather the social factors that impact some minority groups.[4] In this article, the authors examine the prevalence and some identified risk factors for STI in the United States. Specific SDH that have been found to influence the acquisition of STIs and impact the racial disparities that exist are also addressed. Lastly, the long-term impact of SDH and how health care providers can address these factors to reduce STIs are discussed.

THE INCIDENCE AND PREVALENCE OF SEXUALLY TRANSMITTED INFECTIONS IN THE UNITED STATES

Within the last 5 years alone, the incidence and prevalence of STIs has been on the rise. From 2014 to 2018, the number of cases of chlamydia, gonorrhea, and syphilis have increased by 19%, 63%, and 71%, respectively.[5] These statistics are especially concerning given that recently, gonorrhea rates were at an all-time low and syphilis was close to eradication.[5] Much of the previous success was attributed to advances in STI prevention, screening, and diagnostic testing. Although rates of chlamydia, gonorrhea, and syphilis have increased, human immunodeficiency virus (HIV) rates between 2012 and 2016 have remained stable.[6] Although it is important to examine the rates of STIs as a whole, the statistics are variable when factoring in age, sex, race, and ethnicity. Specifically, race and ethnicity are at the core of connecting SDH to STI acquisition rates.

Chlamydia

Chlamydia (*Chlamydia trachomatis*) is the most commonly reported STI in the United States.[7] According to the 2018 STI Surveillance Report, the Centers for Disease Control and Prevention (CDC) reported a total of 1.8 million cases of chlamydia, a 19% increase since 2014.[5] This case count is equivalent to a rate of 539.9 cases per 100,000 population. When examined further, major variations are noted among sex, age, and race (**Table 1**). In 2018, females accounted for 1,145,063 cases of chlamydia, a rate of 692.7 per 100,000 females. Whereas, in the same year, 610,447 cases of chlamydia were reported among males, for a rate of 380.6 cases per 100,000 males. When considering age, the rates of chlamydia are still highest among females. In 2018, females aged 15 to 44 year old accounted for 97.4% of the chlamydia cases, with the highest rates among those aged 15 to 19 and 20 to 24, with rates of 3306.8 and 4064.6 per 100,000 females, respectively. The higher rates among females is also noted when factoring in race. In 2018, the rate of reported chlamydia cases among black females was five times higher than that of white female counterparts with rates of 1411.1 and 281.7 cases per 100,000, respectively.[5] Black males exhibited a similar disparity with a chlamydial rate 6.8 times that of white males.[5]

Gonorrhea

Gonorrhea is among the STI that has seen a dramatic increase in rates. In 2018, there were 583,405 cases reported, a 63% increase since 2014.[5] As noted for chlamydia rates, disparate rates are also noted for gonorrhea (**Table 2**). Unlike chlamydia, the rates of gonorrhea are highest among males. In 2018, the rate of gonorrhea reported was 212.8 cases per 100,000 males and 145.8 cases per 100,000 females, which represented an increase of 78.7% and 45.2%, respectively, from 2014.[5] Gonorrhea showed trends similar to chlamydia with respect to age. Adolescents and young adults ranked among the highest cases for both males and females. Additionally,

Table 1
2018 US chlamydia rates by age, sex, and race

2018 US Chlamydia Rates	Male Rate[a]	Female Rate[a]
Age		
10–14 y	13.6	92.9
15–19 y	959.0	3306.8
20–24 y	**1784.5**	**4064.6**
25–29 y	1134.7	1726.2
30–34 y	651.3	750.2
35–39 y	370.4	363.9
40–44 y	216.5	176.6
45–54 y	115.1	66.0
55–64 y	41.8	18.5
65+ y	7.4	2.3
Race/Hispanic ethnicity		
AI/AN	409.6	1146.3
Asian	102.9	158.4
Blacks	**952.3**	**1411.1**
Hispanics	246.1	541.3
NHOPI	370.4	1033.5
Whites	140.4	281.7
Multirace	131.6	236.6
Total	380.6	692.7

Bolded values display highest rate for males and females based on age and race.
Abbreviations: AI/AN, American Indian and Alaska Native; NHOPI, Native Hawaiian or Other Pacific Islander.
[a] Per 100,000.
Adapted from The Centers for Disease Control and Prevention. Sexually transmitted disease surveillance 2018. https://www.cdc.gov/std/stats18/default.htm Updated August 27, 2019.

the disparity among races is staggering. The rates of gonorrhea among black males was 8.5 times that of white males, and the rates for black females was 6.9 times that of white females.[5]

Syphilis

The CDC reported a 71% increase in the number of cases of primary and secondary syphilis. With a total of 35,063 cases reported in 2018, syphilis has steadily been on the rise.[5] This increase is further compounded by the increase in congenital syphilis, with a total of 1306 cases in 2018, representing a 185% increase from 2014. The rates of reported syphilis are higher among men and has steadily increased since 2000 (**Table 3**). During 2017 to 2018, the rates of reported syphilis among males increased by 11.3%, whereas the rates of females increased by 30.4%. Disparities in syphilis rates also exist for age. The rates are highest among men age 25 to 29 at 55.7 cases per 100,000 and women age 20 to 24 at 10 cases per 100,000. Although the rates for males are higher than their female counterparts for every race, the disparity between black and white males is most notable (see **Table 3**).

Human Immunodeficiency Virus

The national data for HIV reveals that between the years 2012 and 2016, the number of new cases remained fairly stable.[6] In 2017, there was a reported 38,739 new cases of

Table 2
2018 US gonorrhea rates by age, sex, and race

2018 US Gonorrhea Rates	Male Rate[a]	Female Rate[a]
Age		
10–14 y	4.8	21.3
15–19 y	320.5	548.1
20–24 y	**720.9**	**702.6**
25–29 y	674.0	427.2
30–34 y	481.2	248.3
35–39 y	316.1	139.1
40–44 y	200.5	74.3
45–54 y	120.0	28.6
55–64 y	51.3	7.7
65+ y	9.0	1.0
Race/Hispanic ethnicity		
AI/AN	259.3	397.1
Asian	55.0	17.0
Blacks	**674.4**	**433.3**
Hispanics	143.6	87.4
NHOPI	198.6	163.2
Whites	79.6	62.7
Multirace	111.6	77.4

Bolded values display highest rate for males and females based on age and race.
Abbreviations: AI/AN, American Indian and Alaska Native; NHOPI, Native Hawaiian or Other Pacific Islander.
[a] Per 100,000.
Adapted from The Centers for Disease Control and Prevention. Sexually transmitted disease surveillance 2018. https://www.cdc.gov/std/stats18/default.htm Updated August 27, 2019.

HIV. Of those new cases, the highest rates were among men who have sex with men.[6] Among men who have sex with men, the number of new cases were highest among blacks, followed by Hispanic/Latinos, then whites. In 2017, blacks accounted for 43% of HIV diagnoses and Hispanics/Latinos accounted for 26% of diagnoses, despite that they represent 13% and 18% of the population, respectively.[6] Differences in rates among age groups were also present. Adults aged 25 to 34 years represented the highest number of new cases.

INDIVIDUAL-LEVEL RISK FACTORS FOR SEXUALLY TRANSMITTED INFECTIONS

Individual-level risk behaviors were previously considered a major contributor to racial disparities in STI.[8] These risk factors, including the number of sexual partners, condom use, drug use, and participation in anal sex, were believed to have a direct impact on the acquisition of STIs.[8,9] Studies show that these behaviors also vary significantly between different racial groups.[8,9] Newman and Berman[8] provide an example of data retrieved from the Youth Risk Behavior Survey from 2005. When measuring if youth ever had sexual intercourse, were currently sexually active, first sexual encounter before age 13 years, and more than four sexual partners in their lifetime, data suggested that these high-level sexual risk behaviors were higher among black youth than their white counterparts. This, in turn, could provide insight into

Table 3
2018 US primary and secondary syphilis rates by age, sex, race

2018 US Primary and Secondary Syphilis Rates	Male Rate[a]	Female Rate[a]
Age		
10–14 y	0.1	0.2
15–19 y	10.9	4.3
20–24 y	44.6	**10.0**
25–29 y	**55.7**	9.4
30–34 y	45.8	7.5
35–39 y	33.7	5.8
40–44 y	23.9	3.6
45–54 y	19.0	2.0
55–64 y	8.8	0.7
65+ y	1.8	0.1
Race/Hispanic ethnicity		
AI/AN	21.4	**9.8**
Asian	9.1	0.5
Blacks	**49.5**	8.4
Hispanics	22.7	3.1
NHOPI	29.0	3.5
Whites	10.3	1.8
Multirace	16.7	2.2

Bolded values display highest rate for males and females based on age and race.
 Abbreviations: AI/AN, American Indian and Alaska Native; NHOPI, Native Hawaiian or Other Pacific Islander.
 [a] Per 100,000.
 Adapted from The Centers for Disease Control and Prevention. Sexually transmitted disease surveillance 2018. https://www.cdc.gov/std/stats18/default.htm Updated August 27, 2019.

the racial disparity in STIs. However, more recent studies suggest population-level determinants may play a more critical role.[8]

In assessing the risk for acquisition and prevalence of STIs, individual-level risk behavior cannot fully explain the racial disparities that exist.[8] Inconsistencies in the data also support alternative explanations for racial disparities. In the previous example, although black youth were found to have some more sexual risk behaviors than their white peers, they were also found to be more likely to use condoms and less likely to have used drugs or alcohol before their most recent sexual encounter.[8] Furthermore, it has been found that racial disparities persist despite controlling for such risk factors, including partner number, drug and alcohol use, and anal sex.[8,9] These findings suggest that individual-level risk behavior is insufficient in explaining the racial disparities that exist in STIs. Therefore, additional determinants of health should be considered to fully comprehend disparities in STIs.

SOCIAL DETERMINANTS OF HEALTH AND THE ACQUISITION OF SEXUALLY TRANSMITTED INFECTIONS

Similar to the WHO, the CDC described SDH as circumstances associated with the intersection of where people live, learn, work, and play as correlated with health risks and outcomes.[10] SDH are not typically as modifiable as other contributors of health outcomes. Physical, social, and political environments engineer living conditions that can manipulate the health status of populations. Friedman and coworkers[11] asserted SDH, complex and structural in nature, are accountable for most health inequities. These SDH may be challenging to identify, assess, and remedy during routine appointments within the clinical environment. Systematic approaches are essential to recognize health disparities with organized efforts to alleviate their manifestations.

For decades, researchers have disseminated literature acknowledging that chronic illnesses and infectious diseases do not present arbitrarily in populations and genetic predisposition is limited in its influence.[12] Rather, health disparities are often clustered in socially and economically vulnerable populations as a result of poverty, racism, stigma, limited access to health care, and a lack of education.[12] The Office of Disease Prevention and Health Promotion recommended the creation of an operational definition of health disparities to establish goals, prioritize resources, and measure progress.[13] The concept has garnered significant attention necessitating the need for a well-defined meaning to adequately address SDH. The Office of Disease Prevention and Health Promotion asserted the definition be founded on an ethical and human rights framework sought to address health outcomes reflective of societal injustices, by acknowledging the systemic nature of the phenomenon and its affinity for disadvantaged populations.[13] The organization identified "(a) economic stability, (b) education, (c) social and community context, (d) health and health care, and (e) neighborhood and built environment" as SDH.[14] Healthy People used these concepts to construct objectives that address health disparities and increase health equity.[14]

Within the construct of the SDH, multiple factors have been identified as contributors to disparities in STI (**Table 4**). Some factors have direct impacts on acquisition, whereas the impact of others is more indirect. Geographic area and the trends in urbanicity among persons of color, along with poverty, race, and access to health care have been recognized as social factors influencing increased rates and disparities in STIs.

Urbanicity

STIs are similar in inequitable distribution to other health conditions within disenfranchised populations. Oster and colleagues[15] asserted of the 20 million new cases of STIs annually in the United States, individuals of low socioeconomic status are disproportionally impacted. Hogben and Leichliter[3] placed STIs in epidemiologic context, referring to geographic clustering because of social segregation. It is imperative to consider factors related to living conditions and location when assessing for risk factors.

Table 4
Factors impacting the continued increase in sexually transmitted diseases

Social Factors	Individual Factors
Access to sexually transmitted disease prevention and care related to: Drug use Poverty Stigma Unstable housing	Decreased condom use
Cuts to sexually transmitted disease programs at the state and local level	

From New CDC report: STDs continue to rise in the U.S. Press Release: NCHHSTP Newsroom. Centers for Disease Control and Prevention. https://www.cdc.gov/nchhstp/newsroom/2019/2018-STD-surveillance-report-press-release.html. Accessed October 8, 2019.

The US Census Bureau classified urbanized areas as those with a population greater than 50,000.[16] Hogben and Leichliter[3] noted a correlation between physical proximity and carriers of gonorrhea and syphilis. There were more occurrences of these infections in concentrated areas than would occur by chance.[3] Oster and colleagues[15] concluded large central metropolitan areas foster a higher incidence of HIV, herpes simplex virus 2, chlamydia, and hepatitis B. Prevalence of human papillomavirus and hepatitis C did not differ significantly by population or geography. The tendency for persons of color to live in more urban, geographically clustered areas increases exposure and risk to STIs.

Poverty

Health is often negatively impacted by social segregation engineered through poverty. Areas of high poverty are often plagued by unemployment, crime, and substandard educational opportunities.[17] These factors affect environment and behavior working in synergy to influence health. Individuals in poverty may have limited access to healthy foods or safe neighborhoods to engage in physical activity. Low socioeconomic status may influence intimate partner selection, because income affects where individuals live and socialize.[18] Hogben and Leichliter[3] affirmed residential instability resulting from poverty was recognized as a crucial contributor to an influx in HIV rates among blacks. Residential instability, often a result of unstable employment, further diminishes an individual's ability to afford and access health care. Resource deficiency and inequitable resource allocation has been associated with risky sexual behavior, lack of health care, and increased STI rates.[3]

Race

Race is an integral component in investigating implications of social determinants. Cultural norms, behaviors, and attitudes may encourage associated practices within racial groups. Lutfi and colleagues[17] determined STI prevalence is disproportionate when comparing non-Hispanic blacks with non-Hispanic whites.[17] Non-Hispanic blacks were approximately six times more likely than non-Hispanic whites to contract chlamydia and nearly 10 times more likely to be diagnosed with gonorrhea. Data obtained were independent of risky sexual practices. Therefore, results support a notion that societal structures unjustly influence the prevalence of specific STIs. Hogben and Leichliter[3] reached similar conclusions, documenting that blacks with normative sexual behaviors demonstrated rates of syphilis, HIV/AIDS, chlamydia, and gonorrhea 5.4 to 17.8 times the rate of whites and syphilis rates for Latino migrants are two to four times the rate of the US population. In fact, authors asserted when exploring sexual practices of women in the United States, there was little difference between black and white women between the ages of 15 and 44.[3]

Institutionalized racism, manifested by the long-term effects of segregation, has previously been identified as a factor contributing to the disparities in syphilis rates.[3] Individuals face physical and mental health deficits when they are marginalized or encounter stigma or discrimination.[19] Harling and coworkers[18] postulated race confounds STI risk, with documented disparities most significant among women and African Americans. Understanding the underlying social determinants that influence health disparities is essential in reducing disparities.[3] Likewise, recognition of racial and gender differences is necessary to develop practical goals that decrease disparities within these populations.

Health Care Access

Dr Ghebreyesus, General Director of the WHO, recognized the provision of health as a fundamental right for all humans regardless of race, religion, political affiliation, and economic or social position.[19] Despite international efforts, access to health care remains a significant barrier to the attainment of equitable care for all. Lack of health insurance lessens preventive care and is positively correlated with chlamydial infection among youth.[3] Availability of medical insurance, or managed care, does not ensure individuals will be successful in obtaining health care. Physical barriers, such as finances, lack of transportation, or an inability to be excused from employment, may hinder an infected individual from seeking evaluation and treatment. Furthermore, psychosocial barriers, such as stigma and fear related to STIs and the perception of risky sexual behaviors, should be considered.

IMPACT OF SOCIAL DETERMINANTS OF HEALTH AND CURRENT STATE OF REPRODUCTIVE HEALTH

Prevalence rates are rising in the United States. despite concerted efforts to combat STIs. The CDC released STI surveillance data for 2018. The trends identified are concerning. The report indicates that combined cases of syphilis, gonorrhea, and chlamydia reached an all-time high in the United States in 2018.[20] Specifically, from 2017 to 2018 there was a 5% increase in gonorrhea infection and a 3% increase in chlamydia infection.[20] Such large increases from year to year are quite disturbing, especially when considering the long-term impact of STIs. For instance, the CDC announced 115,00 new reports of syphilis infection with a rising trend in congenital syphilis and related infant death. The trend in congenital syphilis rates mirrors that of females aged 15 to 44 with primary or secondary syphilis (**Fig. 1**).[5] Consequently, the number of congenital syphilis cases has more than doubled in the last 4 years and is currently the highest in 20 years.[21] Untreated congenital syphilis can result in skeletal abnormalities, hepatosplenomegaly, sensorineural deafness, and meningitis.[21] In addition to the risk of transmitting syphilis to infants, pregnant women with

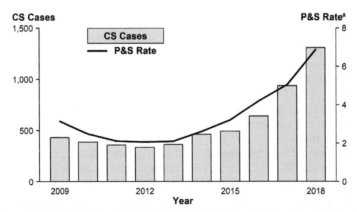

Fig. 1. Congenital syphilis: reported cases by year of birth and rates of reported cases of primary and secondary syphilis among females aged 15 to 44 years, United States, 2009 to 2018. [a] Per 100,000. CS, congenital syphilis; P&S, primary and secondary syphilis. (*From* Centers for Disease Control and Prevention. Sexually transmitted disease surveillance 2018. https://www.cdc.gov/std/stats18/default.htm. Updated August 27, 2019.)

untreated syphilis are at an increased risk for miscarriage and stillbirths.[21] The long-term impact of SDH and STIs is great. Therefore, targeted strategies and interventions are imperative to reduce the increasing rates.

Addressing Social Determinants of Health to Reduce Sexually Transmitted Infections

The CDC identified potential causes for the influx of STI. A list of probable causes included (1) increased drug use, (2) poverty, (3) stigma, (4) housing insecurity, (5) decreased condom use, and (6) a reduction in STI programs.[20] With the exception of reduced condom use, causes identified are categorically classified as SDH. To reduce incidence, strategic programmatic planning must be developed and delivered with intent. Targeted interventions should include culturally appropriate educational strategies specific to disease processes. Braveman and colleagues[13] suggested clinicians become aware of social factors impacting patients and tailor interventions to their home and work environments. The pervasiveness of racial disparities warrants social reform as it relates to marginalized populations. Clinicians are ideal representatives to address health reform and public policy relative to vulnerable populations.

Oster and colleagues[15] postulated recognition of how these populations vary by urbanicity and geography may aid in the creation of more effective interventions. Additional strategies include behavioral health interventions and media campaigns tailored to geographic areas and populations.[15] Interprofessional collaboration and streamlined social work referrals services have been proven to positively impact health outcomes in vulnerable populations.[13] Lastly, Braveman and colleagues[13] acknowledged the importance of further research to explore implications of social construct and health adding to the existing body of evidence.

SUMMARY

There is little debate whether social factors impact health and health status. Social determinants are reflective of the home, work, and community environments. Intangible aspects of social construct, such as education, income, race, access, and social segregation, are equally influential to health outcomes. These dynamics are apparent in consideration of the incidence and prevalence of STI. A call to action is required of clinicians as rates of chlamydia, gonorrhea, and syphilis, once close to eradication, continue to soar. There is promise as rates of HIV continue to show signs of stabilization.

A previous emphasis on prevalence of STI secondary to sexual behaviors and practices is no longer substantiated. Rather, it is crucial to explore population health and determinants to better understand the endemic. Consequently, it is necessary that interventions be tailored to population health and associated social determinants. Initiatives that address race, social segregation, poverty, unemployment, and cultural norms and attitudes may be more effective in creating sustainability within communities. Clinicians should not feel the burden to solve this issue in isolation. Interprofessional collaboration with social workers, policy makers, and researchers can lead to successful patient outcomes.

DISCLOSURE

The authors have nothing to disclose.

REFERENCES

1. About social determinants of health. World Health Organization 2017. Available at: https://www.who.int/social_determinants/sdh_definition/en/. Accessed November 1, 2019.
2. Braveman P, Gottlieb L. The social determinants of health: it's time to consider the causes of the causes. Public Health Rep 2014;129(2):19–31.
3. Hogben M, Leichliter JS. Social determinants and sexually transmitted disease disparities. Sex Transm Dis 2008;35(12):S13–8.
4. STD health equity. Centers for Disease Control and Prevention 2019. Available at: https://www.cdc.gov/std/health-disparities/. Accessed November 1, 2019.
5. Sexually transmitted disease surveillance 2018. Centers for Disease Control and Prevention 2019. Available at: https://www.cdc.gov/std/stats18/default.htm. Accessed November 1, 2019.
6. HIV in the United States and dependent areas. Centers for Disease Control and Prevention 2019. Available at: https://www.cdc.gov/hiv/statistics/overview/ataglance.html. Accessed November 1, 2019.
7. Torrone E, Papp J, Weinstock H. Prevalence of chlamydia trachomatis genital infection among persons aged 14-39 years—United States, 2007-2012. MMWR Morb Mortal Wkly Rep 2014;63(38):834–8.
8. Newman LM, Berman SM. Epidemiology of STD disparities in African American communities. Sex Transm Dis 2008;35(12):S4–12.
9. Hamilton DT, Morris M. The racial disparities in STI: Concurrency, STI prevalence, and heterogeneity in partner selection. Epidemics 2015;11:56–61.
10. Social determinants of health: know what affects health. Centers for Disease Control and Prevention 2018. Available at: https://www.cdc.gov/socialdeterminants/index.htm. Accessed November 1, 2019.
11. Friedman EE, Dean HD, Duffus WA. Incorporation of social determinants of health in the peer-reviewed literature: a systematic review of articles authored by the national center for HIV/AIDS, viral hepatitis, STD, and TB prevention. Public Health Rep 2018;133:392–412.
12. Sharpe TT, Harrison KM, Dean HD. Summary of CDC consultation to address social determinants of health for prevention of disparities in HIV/AIDS, viral hepatitis, sexually transmitted diseases, and tuberculosis. Public Health Rep 2010;125:11–5.
13. Braveman PA, Kumanyika S, Fielding J, et al. Health disparities and health equity: the issue is justice. Am J Public Health 2011;101:149–55.
14. Social Determinants of Health 2019. Available at: https://www.healthypeople.gov/2020/topics-objectives/topic/social-determinants-of-health. Accessed November 1, 2019.
15. Oster AM, Sternberg M, Nebenzahl S, et al. Prevalence of HIV, sexually transmitted infections, and viral hepatitis by urbanicity, among men who have sex with men, injection drug users, and heterosexuals in the United States. Sex Transm Dis 2014;4:272–9.
16. Urban and rural. United States Census Bureau 2018. Available at: https://www.census.gov/programs-surveys/geography/guidance/geo-areas/urban-rural.html. Accessed November 1, 2019.
17. Lutfi K, Trepk MJ, Fennie KP, et al. Racial residential segregation and STI diagnosis among non-Hispanic blacks, 2006–2010. J Immigr Minor Health 2018;20:577–83.

18. Harling G, Subramanian SV, Bärnighausen T, et al. Income inequality and sexually transmitted in the United States: who bears the burden? Soc Sci Med 2014;102: 174–82.

19. Ghebreyesus TA. Health is a fundamental human right: Human Rights Day 2017. World Health Organization. Available at: https://www.who.int/mediacentre/news/statements/fundamental-human-right/en/. Accessed November 1, 2019.

20. New CDC report: STDs continue to rise in the U.S. Press Release: NCHHSTP Newsroom. Centers for Disease Control and Prevention. Available at: https://www.cdc.gov/nchhstp/newsroom/2019/2018-STD-surveillance-report-press-release.html. Accessed November 1, 2019.

21. Bachman LH. A devastating surge in congenital syphilis: how can we stop it? Medscape. Available at: https://www.medscape.com/viewarticle/907183?pa=OExvQildaGyiM25hsXJ2jdL2Kg1m%2FrdRrrApQH%2BVX3sjl6K3vaxz7IHiMK ZUS7P9X8MwC0EECwzp432Skuf9qw%3D%3D. Accessed November 1, 2019.

The Stigma of Sexually Transmitted Infections

Amy S.D. Lee, DNP, ARNP, WHNP-BC*, Shameka L. Cody, PhD, AGNP-C

KEYWORDS

- Stigma • Sexually transmitted infections • Partner treatment • Delayed care
- Provider-patient relationship

KEY POINTS

- A review of the recommendations for screening, diagnosis, and treatment of sexually transmitted infections (STIs) helps identify the issues, challenges, and controversies surrounding the stigma of STIs.
- STI stigma is a barrier to prevention and treatment of STIs.
- STI prevention and STI stigma reduction can be promoted through an understanding of STI detection, treatment, and barriers to care.

INTRODUCTION

The Centers for Disease Control and Prevention (CDC) staff and workgroup members composed of representative experts from the public and private sector released the latest "Sexually Transmitted Disease Treatment Guidelines" updated as of 2015.[1] These guidelines detail treatment and clinical management of sexually transmitted infections (STIs) based on scientific evidence. The evidence-based treatment guidelines have been reviewed by a second independent expert panel to ensure the most accurate data. STIs have been categorized by the CDC into groups with diagnostic and treatment considerations detailed under each category.[1] Through a review of the recommendations for screening, diagnosis, and treatment of each STI, the issues, challenges, and controversies surrounding the stigma of STIs can be identified and further examined.

Even with the shift of terminology from sexually transmitted disease (STD) to sexual transmitted infection (STI), stigma remains a barrier to prevention and treatment.[2] Stigma is defined as an individual's fear that he or she will be subject to negative societal attitudes and treatment based on a specific trait.[3] Some sexual minority populations are more susceptible to experiencing stigma, which contributes to mental

Capstone College of Nursing, The University of Alabama, 650 University Boulevard East, Tuscaloosa, AL 35401, USA
* Corresponding author.
E-mail address: adlee5@ua.edu

Nurs Clin N Am 55 (2020) 295–305
https://doi.org/10.1016/j.cnur.2020.05.002
0029-6465/20/© 2020 Elsevier Inc. All rights reserved.

health issues, increased risky behaviors, and underutilization of STI health care services.[4] Sociodemographic and structural factors are important in identifying high-risk groups likely to underutilize STI preventative services. However, stigma in the clinical setting, including provider-patient relationship issues, can discourage STI testing and disclosure of symptoms. Combined factors or multilayer stigma effects may further delay STI testing and partner notification, both of which can lead to greater STI outbreaks.[3] Some infected individuals who encounter STI-associated stigma may not notify their partner and fail to return for follow-up treatment. Similarly, some uninfected individuals who face STI-associated stigma may delay testing, which can be detrimental, especially if they have sexual contact with a known infected partner. The key to STI prevention and reducing stigma is to understand what contributes to underutilization of health care services.[4] Interdisciplinary researchers and health care providers have a shared role in promoting culturally sensitive sexual health language and increasing provider competence to optimize care for unique high-risk populations.

SEXUALLY TRANSMITTED INFECTIONS REVIEW
Human Immunodeficiency Virus

Human immunodeficiency virus (HIV) begins as a brief acute retroviral syndrome that culminates in life-threatening immunodeficiency known as AIDS.[1] Diagnosis during the acute phase is critical to effective treatment and prevention because the early phase is highly infectious. All patients seeking routine care for STI screening or STIs should be screened for HIV. HIV is diagnosed through serologic tests that undergo confirmatory secondary testing if repeatedly positive. With the availability of effective antiretroviral therapy, a patient with HIV today can expect to live a normal lifespan. Counseling and support services should be provided. Partner notification is important and should be facilitated by the health care provider.[1]

Ulcerative Diseases

Prevalence of sexually transmitted genital ulcerative lesions is affected by geographic area and population, but the most commonly seen in the United States are genital herpes and syphilis, with herpes seen most frequently.[1] Genital ulcerative lesions are a risk factor for the acquisition and transmission of HIV.[1]

Genital herpes is a chronic life-long recurring infection caused by either herpes simplex virus (HSV) type I or type II. Most genital herpes are caused by HSV type II, but genital HSV type I prevalence has increased. Most people with the infection are unaware of the diagnosis. Therefore, the virus intermittently sheds without awareness because of either very mild symptoms or asymptomatic shedding of the virus. It is important to counsel the patient on the chronicity of the infection with the potential for infection of others throughout life. Direct cell culture and polymerase chain reaction assay testing (DNA testing) of the active lesion is the preferred testing source. Serologic testing may be completed that will determine if HSV I or II antibodies are present. Treatment with systemic oral antiviral medications can be initiated on suspicion of genital herpes while awaiting diagnostic confirmation. It should be noted that antivirals reduce symptoms and shedding but do not eradicate the virus. All new patients with an HSV diagnosis should be tested for HIV and counseled/supported regarding the implications of the infection.[1]

Syphilis is a systemic infection caused by the bacteria Treponema pallidum.[1] There are 4 stages of syphilis infection starting with the primary stage heralded by an ulcerative lesion or chancre. The secondary stage sees resolution of the ulcerative lesion and progression to skin rash, mucocutaneous lesions, and lymphadenopathy, whereas the tertiary stage is characterized by cardiac, gummatous lesions, tabes dorsalis, and general paresis. The latent stage occurs if syphilis goes undiagnosed, during which time the central nervous system may become infected, resulting in neurosyphilis. It is thought that syphilis is transmitted only when mucocutaneous lesions are present, and these are generally only seen in the first year after contracting the disease. Diagnosis of syphilis requires both a treponemal and a nontreponemal test for confirmation. Nontreponemal antibody titers can be used to monitor treatment response and are useful in detecting reexposure in previously positive/treated people. Parenteral penicillin G is used to effectively treat and prevent the sequelae of syphilis. Treatment regimens are prolonged for those with latent syphilis. All patients diagnosed with syphilis should be tested for HIV.[1]

Urethritis, Cervicitis, Vaginal Discharge

Mycoplasma genitalium is a bacterial infection that may be responsible for urethral inflammation and cervicitis that can be sexually transmitted.[1] Currently, there are no Food and Drug Administration (FDA)-approved tests in the United States for *M genitalium*. Consideration for presumptive treatment of patient and partners with antimicrobials should be given after repeated recurrence and exclusion of other causes.[1]

Chlamydia trachomatis or chlamydia is the most commonly reported infection in the United States with the highest prevalence in those individuals under the age of 25 years.[1] Although asymptomatic infection is common in women and men, significant long-term chlamydia sequelae for women include ectopic pregnancy, pelvic inflammatory disease, and infertility. Routine screening through urine, vaginal, or cervical nuclei acid amplification (NAAT) sampling for chlamydia is recommended annually in all women under the age of 25 and in women over the age of 25 with risk factors for infection (new partner, >1 partner, partner with other partner, exposure to partner with known STI).[1,5] Self-swab vaginal and rectal swab collection has been found to be comparable to clinician collected and often more preferable for the patient. Patients and partners should be treated with a recommended antimicrobial regimen.[1] Expedited partner treatment (EPT) has been shown to be an effective option for partner treatment whereby partners may be provided a prescription or the medications, but EPT allowability is regulated by state law and varies from state to state.[5] STI retesting should be undertaken 3 months after treatment because of high reinfection rates.[1]

Neisseria gonorrhoeae or gonorrhea is the second most common communicable disease reported in the United States.[1] Symptoms are often initially so vague that detection occurs too late to prevent transmission or complications (eg, pelvic inflammatory disease, tubal scarring). Such complications result in infertility and ectopic pregnancy risk. Routine screening through urine, vaginal, or cervical NAAT or culture sampling for gonorrhea is recommended annually in all women under the age of 25, in women over the age of 25 with increased risk for infection, or in men of any age with increased risk for infection. Because of *N gonorrhoeae*'s ability to develop antimicrobial resistance, it is important to treat both patients and their partners with recommended antimicrobials on site under the observation of the health care team.[1] Again, EPT has been shown to be an effective treatment option depending on state allowability.[5] Retesting should be completed in 3 months because of the high rate of reinfection. Those positive for gonorrhea should be screened fully for other STIs.[1]

Trichomoniasis vaginalis, the most common nonviral STI in the United States, is characterized by urethritis in men and malodorous yellow-green vaginal discharge in women.[1] However, it can often be asymptomatic. It is highly transmissible through penile-vaginal intercourse and increases the risk of HIV transmission 2- to 3-fold as well as preterm birth and pregnancy complications. Wet-mount preparations, culture, and NAAT testing can be undertaken to diagnose trichomoniasis, but NAAT testing has been shown to be significantly more sensitive. Nitroimidazoles are the only antimicrobial class shown to effectively treat trichomoniasis. Both the patient and any partners should be treated and should abstain from intercourse until treatment is complete and symptoms have abated, and retesting in 3 months should be completed. The patient should be screened for all other STIs, including HIV.[1]

Bacterial vaginosis (BV) is a polymicrobial syndrome caused by the replacement of the normal vaginal Lactobacillus with anaerobic bacteria.[1] BV is seen more commonly in those women who have multiple partners, new partners, or sex without condoms. Although it has not been found to be related to any particular sexually transmitted pathogen, women with BV have been found to be at higher risk for other STIs. Treatment can be achieved with oral or vaginal antimicrobial therapy. Treatment of sexual partners is not recommended. Follow-up is not necessary if symptoms resolve, although BV will often recur.[1]

Human Papilloma Virus

There are about 100 identified subtypes of the human papilloma virus (HPV) with around 40 of them capable of infecting the genital area.[1] Most of these infections are self-limiting. However, certain oncogenic high-risk subtypes are responsible for most cervical, penile, vulvar, vaginal, anal, and oropharyngeal cancers. There are several HPV vaccines available in the United States that offer protection from the highest-risk subtypes. The vaccine is recommended for girls and boys by age 11 or 12 but may be given as early as age 9. HPV tests are available for women in conjunction with cervical cytology screening or management for oncogenic subtype detection.[1] There are currently no available tests for oropharyngeal HPV.[6] Testing of partners is not indicated. Most subclinical infections clear spontaneously and do not require treatment. However, persistent infection with oncogenic subtypes is the greatest risk factor for the development of HPV-associated cancers. Treatment is therefore directed at management of dysplastic lesions or visible warts.[1]

Viral Hepatitis

Hepatitis A is a viral infection that replicates in the liver and is commonly spread through the fecal/oral route.[1] Any sexual transmission is thought to be through fecal contact. The infection is self-limiting and does not result in chronic infection or chronic liver disease. The most effective form of prevention is through vaccination. Treatment is supportive.

Hepatitis B is a viral infection that is transmitted through blood and body fluids.[1] Sexual transmission is the most common source of hepatitis B transmission in the United States.[7] It may be self-limiting or become a chronic infection. The risk for premature death owing to hepatocellular carcinoma or cirrhosis is 15% to 25% for those chronically infected. Because there is no curative treatment, prevention through vaccination is critical. Vaccination is recommended routinely for infants or any older child or adult who has not been vaccinated. Treatment of those infected is supportive.[1]

Hepatitis C is a blood-borne viral infection of the liver that can be sexually transmitted but is not commonly transmitted this way.[7] However, those with a history of STIs, HIV, multiple sex partners, or "rough sex" are shown to have a higher risk of contracting hepatitis C. Hepatitis C may be self-limiting, but 70% to 85% of those infected will develop chronic infection with risk of long-term health problems, including death.[8] There is no vaccine for hepatitis C.[1] However, significant advances in treatment of hepatitis C have allowed for complete cure of hepatitis C in those with chronic infection.[9]

Ectoparasitic Infections

Pediculosis pubis (pubic lice) and scabies are transmitted through sexual contact.[1] Most patients present for care because of pruritis or visible lice. Treatment is through topical creams or lotions. Treatment of partners and decontamination of bedding and living spaces are required[1] (**Table 1**).

SEXUALLY TRANSMITTED INFECTIONS STIGMA AND CONTROVERSIES
Stigma and Treatment of Sexually Transmitted Infections

The ability to express one's health concerns to health care providers remains a challenge and an important step to early STI diagnosis. Negative health care climates are known to influence health-seeking behaviors and may even hinder infected individuals from referring their partners for treatment. Some of the reported attitudes of health care providers include inattentiveness to health care needs and expressing disapproval of sexual behaviors contributing to diagnosis and/or reinfection.[10] Studies have found greater social stigmatization associated with viral STIs compared with bacterial STIs that are easily treated with antibiotics.[11] Even with reassurance of health care providers, some individuals fear disclosure of their STI. Unintentional disclosure is possible if someone sees them at an STI clinic. Also, a request to return to the clinic often means a positive test result that warrants treatment. Once an individual receives notification of a positive test result, they may delay or refuse to seek treatment in fear that others may find out about their diagnosis.[12] The fear of STI disclosure can be more problematic especially for those who wish to conceal their sexual identity. Long clinic wait times are associated with greater fear of unintentional disclosure of STI, and for a gay man, concerns that others will suspect he has HIV.[10] Rather than risk breach of confidentiality and/or encounter subsequent stigma in the clinical setting, many choose to use over-the-counter medications to manage STI symptoms.[10]

In addition, internal stigma or self-stigmatization refers to the shame of one's own behavior and expected discrimination that prevents them from seeking treatment.[13] Internal stigma has been shown to impact perceptions of sexual risk and health-seeking behaviors.[13] When people demonstrate self-blame and guilt, they may be reluctant to seek treatment and think that a diagnosis of an STI is a consequence of their sexual behavior and same-sex preferences. Societal stigma coupled with internal stigma can lessen adherence to treatment and clinic visits.[13] Psychological distress commonly occurs with an STI diagnosis, and without cotreatment of such distress, there is a risk of medication resistance and increased risky behaviors.[14]

Alternatives for Sexually Transmitted Infection Testing

The pelvic examination and urethral swab are standard methods for gonorrhea and chlamydia screening in the clinical setting, and such invasive procedures are considered barriers to routine testing among high-risk populations.[15] Noninvasive screening for these 2 common STIs includes urine specimen collection and self-obtained vaginal swabs.[15] Although these methods lessen discomfort, in-home STI screening has been explored to improve confidentiality and stigma faced in the clinic setting.[16] Individuals who are difficult to reach for STI testing may be more willing to perform testing in the privacy of their own home. Studies found vaginal swabs were preferable for women because of tedious packaging and storage of urine samples.[17] STI-related stigma is

Table 1
Various sexually transmitted infection reviews

STI	Cause	Diagnosis	Treatment	Partner Notification?
HIV	Viral	Serologic	Antiretroviral, not curative	Yes
HSV	Viral	Direct NAAT, serologic	Antiretroviral, not curative	Yes
Syphilis	Bacterial	Serologic	Antimicrobial	Yes
M genitalium	Bacterial	Symptomatic, no FDA approved	Antimicrobial	Yes
Chlamydia (CT)	Bacterial	Direct NAAT	Antimicrobial	Yes
Gonorrhea (GC)	Bacterial	Direct NAAT	Antimicrobial	Yes
Trichomonas	Parasite	Wet prep, direct NAAT, culture	Antimicrobial	Yes
Bacterial vaginosis	Bacterial	Wet prep	Antimicrobial	No
HPV	Viral	Pap, HPV specific	None, vaccination	No
Hepatitis A	Viral	Serologic	None, vaccination	No
Hepatitis B	Viral	Serologic	None, vaccination	Yes
Hepatitis C	Viral	Serologic	Targeted antiviral, cure possible	Yes
Ectoparasitic	Parasite	Visual	Creams, decontamination	Yes

still problematic for individuals who need follow-up treatment after performing in-home testing. Other solutions, such as e-medicine, are more convenient than coming into a clinic for treatment. However, many of these services are costly, and insurance copays vary for medications called in to a local pharmacy.

Similarly, researchers examined the impact of HIV self-testing on routine screening and STI risk. In a recent study, Katz and colleagues[18] randomized 230 HIV-negative men who have sex to a control group that underwent HIV testing over 15 months in the clinic or an intervention group trained to perform an in-home monthly oral HIV test. They found that men in the intervention group reported significantly more frequent HIV testing during follow-up compared with those in the control group. In addition, most of them thought they would self-test 4 or more times per year if the test cost $5 or less.[18] Although cost of self-testing kits may be another barrier to routine screening, HIV self-testing has the potential to reach individuals who have never been tested and those who test infrequently. If an individual has a positive HIV result from in-home testing, confirmatory testing in the clinical setting may be recommended with prompt initiation of antiretroviral therapy. Given this, HIV testing in the home may be avoided if there is fear of a positive result, especially if follow-up treatment is expected to take place in a clinic setting. Prompt linkage to care may be less likely with in-home HIV testing compared with clinic testing, and the ability to detect early HIV infection with self-testing warrants further study.[18]

State Mandated Sexually Transmitted Infection Screening

According to the CDC, congenital syphilis rates increased from 8.4 to 15.7 cases per 100,000 live births, representing an 87% increase in the United States from 2012 to

2016.[19] State laws related to syphilis screening during pregnancy vary with some states having penalties for providers who fail to screen pregnant mothers for syphilis.[20] Warren and colleagues[20] found that 6 states among the United States and DC do not require prenatal syphilis screening, and of the 45 remaining states that require prenatal screening, the timeframe for testing during pregnancy varied and penalties for providers who failed to administer a prenatal syphilis test included criminal misdemeanor, civil penalty, and license revocation. The rates of prenatal syphilis screening are likely to be higher for states in which there are penalties for not screening. However, the prenatal screening requirements for some states allow a woman to refuse testing.[20] Unfortunately, some pregnant women who lack adequate prenatal care may have a higher risk of congenital syphilis. From 2008 to 2014, women who did not have access to prenatal care comprised 21.8% of the congenital syphilis cases.[21] Disparities in prenatal care and variations in state screening guidelines need further investigation to determine how such factors impact prevalence rates in the United States.

Adolescents Seeking Care for Sexually Transmitted Infections

Stigma and lack of confidentiality have been identified as barriers to adolescents accessing care for STIs. Newton-Levinson and colleagues[22] found system-specific barriers, such as lack of integration of STI care, with other services, such as maternal health, primary care, and family planning, created concerns about confidentiality among youth seeking care for STIs at specialized clinics. Several studies have suggested primary care providers offer STI testing services for convenience and to increase screening among youth without fear of stigma.[23] In a study of 198 men who have sex with men aged 14 to 17 years, more than 50% avoided communicating their sexual orientation and sexual health concerns to providers because of fear of heterosexist bias, fear of disclosure of their sexual orientation to their parents, and belief that sexual minority youth do not receive equitable treatment in health care settings.[24] Other issues with adolescents seeking care for STIs relate to perception of screening and knowledge of consequences of untreated STIs.[23] Some adolescents value STI screening to reassure them of their partner's status and confirm fidelity in their relationships. Also, they may be ashamed to have STI testing if the provider is older, because it would feel like their parent was present. Some studies have shown that adolescents avoid STI screening with older providers because they are insensitive, are judgmental, and often scold them for their sexual behavior.[23] Social stigma is a barrier given that some adolescents believe their identity would be compromised if they needed to get tested.

Ethical Issues Related to Vaccinations

Uptake of human papillomavirus (HPV) vaccination in the United States is relatively low despite its high efficacy in reducing risk of cervical, anal, and genital cancers.[25,26] In 2017, only 68.6% of young women and 62.6% of young men had initiated the vaccine sequence in the United States, whereas only 53.1% of young women and 44.3% of young men had received all of the recommended doses.[24,25] Some parents are concerned that HPV vaccination may encourage adolescents to engage in risky sexual behaviors in the future. However, several studies have shown that HPV vaccination is not predictive of subsequent sexual behaviors among adolescents and young adults.[25,27,28] Prior studies in girls and women have shown no difference in those vaccinated and unvaccinated in regards to the number of sexual partners,[29] diagnosis of pregnancy or STI,[30] contraception counseling,[31] and condom use and the number of girls who were sexually active.[32] Mullins and colleagues[28] found that adolescents were more likely to use condoms if their mother communicated with them about the

HPV vaccine, which suggests that parent-child communication can facilitate reduced sexual health risks and STI prevention.

Vaccination for hepatitis B, a viral infection transmitted through exposure to infected blood or mucous membranes, has been recommended and mandated in most states in the United States.[33] Today, almost all states require the hepatitis B 3-dose series for preschool and K-12 school attendance. Parents are concerned about potential adverse reactions (eg, neurodevelopmental disorders) from the hepatitis B vaccine that far outweigh their child's risk of hepatitis B infection.[34] Interventions to prevent transmission of hepatitis B from mother to child produce ethical concerns for patients with certain religious beliefs as well.[35] Health care providers should always consider what is mandated by their state, the family's religious beliefs, and what is in the best interest for the child.

Ethical Issues Related to Partner Services

The goal of partner services is to increase HIV awareness, improve linkage to care, increase disease surveillance, and decrease HIV incidence rates in the community.[36] Individuals with an STI and their partner can benefit from an array of services, including prevention counseling and testing for other types of STIs, hepatitis screening and vaccination, and prompt referral and linkage to care if diagnosed with HIV. Some patients feel comfortable referring their sex/drug injection partner or partners for STI screening on their own, whereas others prefer health care providers assist with notifying their partner. This process can be difficult for some newly diagnosed patients if they are worried that their partner will suspect infidelity and if there is a risk of intimate partner violence. Some clinics participate in partner notification and treatment therapy programs in which the patient is treated and given an additional dose or prescription of the medication to take to their partner. Although this may reduce the risk of reinfection and remove the inconvenience of STI clinic screening for the partner, some patients still fear their partner's reaction when they disclose their STI diagnosis. John and colleagues[37] examined 196 patient surveys and found that nearly one-third were worried about intimate partner violence when delivering medication to their partner for an STI. Qualitative interviews revealed concerns of possible arguments with their partners that may lead to physical fights, jail time, or even murder.[37] These conversations are difficult to initiate, and health care providers should prepare patients to discuss their diagnosis with their partners. Intimate partner violence can be traumatic for patients, and in the worst cases, patients may fail to inform their partners and/or fail to notify police of violent incidents because of distrust and fear of retaliation.

Criminalization of Human Immunodeficiency Virus Exposure

HIV criminalization is another barrier to HIV testing. Several states have penalties for individuals diagnosed with HIV who engage in sexual activity with others without disclosing their HIV status.[38] Whether HIV criminalization contributes to the increasing number of undiagnosed HIV cases remains uncertain. HIV exposure laws are designed to decrease prevalence of new infections and encourage individuals diagnosed with HIV to engage in safer sex practices. However, in a sample of 479 people living with HIV, Galletly and colleagues[39] found that awareness of the HIV exposure law was not associated with increased sexual abstinence, condom use, or disclosure of seropositive status. Galletly and colleagues[39] also found that awareness of the exposure law reduced stigma for people living with HIV but it did not likely reduce transmission of the disease (**Box 1**).

Box 1
Sexually transmitted infections stigma issues

- Delayed or deferred testing and treatment
- Testing-related issues and barriers
- State-mandated screening inconsistencies
- Adolescent privacy
- Vaccination concerns
- Partner notification and treatment
- HIV criminalization

SUMMARY

Knowledge and understanding of STIs help identify the issues and controversies contributing to the stigma created by STI diagnosis, management, and treatment. The CDC provides a thorough and complete discussion of STIs that allow the health care team to gain the necessary understanding of the underlying factors surrounding STI stigma.[1] STI stigma in the clinical setting can lead to resistance to STI testing, avoidance of symptom disclosure, and overall delay in diagnosis and treatment. The provider-patient relationship may contribute to reluctance in screening, whereas other combined factors may further delay STI testing and partner notification. A delay in diagnosis or inadequate partner notification easily results in increased STI cases and resulting morbidity.[3]

The key to STI prevention and reducing stigma is to understand the contributing factors.[4] A thorough understanding of STI symptoms, diagnosis, management, and treatment illuminates those factors that help create the stigma associated with STIs. Furthermore, examining the underutilization of health care services and seeking to overcome these barriers promote STI prevention and reduces the stigma of STIs.[4]

DISCLOSURE

The authors have nothing to disclose.

REFERENCES

1. Center for Disease Control and Prevention (CDC). 2015 sexually transmitted diseases treatment guidelines. Available at: https://www.cdc.gov/std/tg2015/tg-2015-print.pdf. Accessed December 6, 2019.
2. Lederer AM, Laing EE. What's in a name? Perceptions of the terms sexually transmitted disease and sexually transmitted infection among late adolescents. Sex Transm Dis 2017;44(11):707–11.
3. Morris JL, Lippman SA, Philip S, et al. Sexually transmitted infection related stigma and shame among African American male youth: implications for testing practices, partner notification, and treatment. AIDS Patient Care STDS 2014; 28(9):499–506.
4. Winskell K, Sabben G. Sexual stigma and symbolic violence experienced, enacted, and counteracted in young Africans' writing about same-sex attraction. Soc Sci Med 2016;161:143–50.
5. Pickett ML, Goyal MK. Diagnosis and treatment of sexually transmitted infections in the emergency department. Clin Pediatr Emerg Med 2019;20(1):4–8.

6. Katz A. CE: Human papillomavirus-related oral cancers: the nurse's role in mitigating stigma and dispelling myths. Am J Nurs 2017;117(1):34–9.
7. Sexual transmission and viral hepatitis | populations and settings | division of viral hepatitis | CDC. Available at: https://www.cdc.gov/hepatitis/populations/stds.htm. Accessed December 6, 2019.
8. Center for Disease Control and Prevention (CDC). Hepatitis C information | division of viral hepatitis | CDC. Available at: https://www.cdc.gov/hepatitis/hcv/index.htm. Accessed December 6, 2019.
9. Center for Disease Control and Prevention (CDC). Hepatitis C questions and answers for health professionals | CDC. Available at: https://www.cdc.gov/hepatitis/hcv/hcvfaq.htm. Accessed December 6, 2019.
10. Kushwaha S, Lalani Y, Maina G, et al. "But the moment they find out that you are MSM …": a qualitative investigation of HIV prevention experiences among men who have sex with men (MSM) in Ghana's health care system. BMC Public Health 2017;17(1). https://doi.org/10.1186/s12889-017-4799-1.
11. Swamiappan M, Chandran V, Prabhakar P. A retrospective study of the pattern of sexually transmitted infections in males: viral infections in emerging trend. J Clin Diagn Res 2016;10(1):WC01–3.
12. UNAIDS. Confronting discrimination: overcoming HIV-related stigma and discrimination in healthcare settings and beyond. Geneva (Switzerland): UNAIDS; 2017. Available at: https://www.unaids.org/sites/default/files/media_asset/confronting-discrimination_en.pdf.
13. Pantelic M, Sprague L, Stangl AL. It's not "all in your head": critical knowledge gaps on internalized HIV stigma and a call for integrating social and structural conceptualizations. BMC Infect Dis 2019;19(1). https://doi.org/10.1186/s12879-019-3704-1.
14. Shubber Z, Mills EJ, Nachega JB, et al. Patient-reported barriers to adherence to antiretroviral therapy: a systematic review and meta-analysis. PLoS Med 2016; 13(11). https://doi.org/10.1371/journal.pmed.1002183.
15. Graseck AS, Shih SL, Peipert JF. Home versus clinic-based specimen collection for Chlamydia trachomatis and Neisseria gonorrhoeae. Expert Rev Anti Infect Ther 2011;9(2):183–94.
16. Habel MA, Scheinmann R, Verdesoto E, et al. Exploring pharmacy and home-based sexually transmissible infection testing. Sex Health 2015;12(6):472–9.
17. Taylor D, Lunny C, Wong T, et al. Self-collected versus clinician-collected sampling for sexually transmitted infections: a systematic review and meta-analysis protocol. Syst Rev 2013;2:93.
18. Katz DA, Golden MR, Hughes JP, et al. HIV self-testing increases HIV testing frequency in high-risk men who have sex with men: a randomized controlled trial. J Acquir Immune Defic Syndr 2018;78:505–12.
19. Center for Disease Control and Prevention (CDC). Syphilis–2018 sexually transmitted diseases surveillance. Available at: https://www.cdc.gov/std/stats18/syphilis.htm. Accessed December 6, 2019.
20. Warren HP, Cramer R, Kidd S, et al. State requirements for prenatal syphilis screening in the United States, 2016. Matern Child Health J 2018;22(9):1227–32.
21. Bowen V, Su J, Torrone E, et al. Increase in incidence of congenital syphilis–United States, 2012-2014. Morb Mortal Wkly Rep 2015;64(44):1241–5.
22. Newton-Levinson A, Leichliter JS, Chandra-Mouli V. Sexually transmitted infection services for adolescents and youth in low- and middle-income countries: perceived and experienced barriers to accessing care. J Adolesc Health 2016; 59(1):7–16.

23. Normansell R, Drennan VM, Oakeshott P. Exploring access and attitudes to regular sexually transmitted infection screening: the views of young, multi-ethnic, inner-city, female students. Health Expect 2016;19(2):322–30.
24. Fisher CB, Fried AL, Macapagal K, et al. Patient–provider communication barriers and facilitators to HIV and STI preventive services for adolescent MSM. AIDS Behav 2018;22(10):3417–28.
25. Brouwer AF, Delinger RL, Eisenberg MC, et al. HPV vaccination has not increased sexual activity or accelerated sexual debut in a college-aged cohort of men and women. BMC Public Health 2019;19(1). https://doi.org/10.1186/s12889-019-7134-1.
26. Walker TY, Elam-Evans LD, Yankey D, et al. National, regional, state, and selected local area vaccination coverage among adolescents aged 13–17 years—United States, 2017. MMWR Morb Mortal Wkly Rep 2018;67(33):909–17.
27. Kornides ML, McRee AL, Gilkey MB. Parents who decline HPV vaccination: who later accepts and why? Acad Pediatr 2018;18(2):S37–43.
28. Mullins TLK, Zimet GD, Rosenthal SL, et al. Human papillomavirus vaccine-related risk perceptions and subsequent sexual behaviors and sexually transmitted infections among vaccinated adolescent women. Vaccine 2016;34(34): 4040–5.
29. Hansen BT, Kjær SK, Arnheim-Dahlström L, et al. Human papillomavirus (HPV) vaccination and subsequent sexual behaviour: evidence from a large survey of Nordic women. Vaccine 2014;32(39):4945–53.
30. Smith LM, Kaufman JS, Strumpf EC, et al. Effect of human papillomavirus (HPV) vaccination on clinical indicators of sexual behaviour among adolescent girls: the Ontario Grade 8 HPV Vaccine Cohort Study. CMAJ 2015;187(2):E74–81.
31. Bednarczyk RA, Davis R, Ault K, et al. Sexual activity-related outcomes after human papillomavirus vaccination of 11- to 12-year-olds. Pediatrics 2012;130(5): 798–805.
32. Forster AS, Marlow LAV, Stephenson J, et al. Human papillomavirus vaccination and sexual behaviour: cross-sectional and longitudinal surveys conducted in England. Vaccine 2012;30(33):4939–44.
33. Schillie S, Harris A, Link-Gelles R, et al. Recommendations of the advisory committee on immunization practices for use of a hepatitis B vaccine with a novel adjuvant. Morb Mortal Wkly Rep 2018;67(15):455–8.
34. The flawed logic of hepatitis B vaccine mandates. Available at: https://www. theepochtimes.com/the-flawed-logic-of-hepatitis-b-vaccine-mandates_2788590. html. Accessed December 6, 2019.
35. Isaacs D, Kilham HA, Alexander S, et al. Ethical issues in preventing mother-to-child transmission of hepatitis B by immunisation. Vaccine 2011;29(37):6159–62.
36. Rorie M, Song W, Zhang H, et al. Partner Services 2016 Report Highlights. Atlanta (GA): Centers for Disease Control and Prevention; 2018. Available at: https:// stacks.cdc.gov/view/cdc/58348.
37. John SA, Walsh JL, Cho YI, et al. Perceived risk of intimate partner violence among STI clinic patients: implications for partner notification and patient-delivered partner therapy. Arch Sex Behav 2018;47(2):481–92.
38. Lehman JS, Carr MH, Nichol AJ, et al. Prevalence and public health implications of state laws that criminalize potential HIV exposure in the United States. AIDS Behav 2014;18(6):997–1006.
39. Galletly CL, Glasman LR, Pinkerton SD, et al. New Jersey's HIV exposure law and the HIV-related attitudes, beliefs, and sexual and seropositive status disclosure behaviors of persons living with HIV. Am J Public Health 2012;102(11):2135–40.

Update on Guidelines for Sexually Transmitted Infection Treatment and Management in the Adult and Adolescent Population

Anna Richmond, DNP, FNP-C, PNP-PC[a],*,
Mary Lauren Pfieffer, DNP, FNP-BC, CPN[b],
Queen Henry-Okafor, PhD, FNP-BC, PMHNP-BC[b]

KEYWORDS

- Sexually transmitted infections • STIs • STI treatment • STI guidelines
- STI primary care

KEY POINTS

- Sexually transmitted infection (STI) treatment is changing frequently and providers need to remain current on guidelines for treatment.
- STIs are a public health concern and swift treatment is key to decreasing the spread of infection.
- Patient education on treatment and prevention therapies is a key component to controlling the spread of STIs.

INTRODUCTION

Sexually transmitted infections (STIs) are a prevalent global health care problem. Incidence rates are rising yearly.[1] STI incidence is highest for adolescents and young adults ages 15 to 24 years, as they are diagnosed with half of all new STIs.[1] *Chlamydia trachomatis* and *Neisseria gonorrhea* are common STIs caused by bacteria.[1]

Prompt treatment is necessary for successful eradication of infection and decreased partner transmission. Treatment of STIs should focus on providing effective, well-tolerated treatment given in as few doses as possible. The condensed treatment improves medication adherence and treatment success. Patient education regarding medication specifics and sexual abstinence during treatment aids in STI

[a] Vanderbilt University School of Nursing, 356 Frist Hall, 461 21st Avenue South, Nashville, TN 37240, USA; [b] Vanderbilt University School of Nursing, 354 Frist Hall, 461 21st Avenue South, Nashville, TN 37240, USA
* Corresponding author.
E-mail address: anna.richmond@vanderbilt.edu

Nurs Clin N Am 55 (2020) 307–323
https://doi.org/10.1016/j.cnur.2020.06.001
0029-6465/20/© 2020 Elsevier Inc. All rights reserved.

nursing.theclinics.com

eradication. STIs are differentiated as bacterial or viral but their treatment is pathogen-specific.

BACTERIAL INFECTIONS
Chlamydia trachomatis

Chlamydia trachomatis is a common STI caused by bacteria.[1] *Chlamydia trachomatis* is highly susceptible to antibiotics like tetracyclines and macrolides. When possible, directly observed single-dose therapy should be administered to patients if adherence is a concern.[2] In some states, health care providers can write a prescription for partners without examining them, referred to as expedited partner therapy or patient-delivered partner therapy. The Centers for Disease Control and Prevention (CDC) also recommends administering the first dose of 7-day regimens by direct observation, if available. See **Table 1** for dosing.

Patients should be counseled to avoid sexual contact for 7 days after treatment with single-dose therapy or until completion of a 7-day therapy and resolution of symptoms.[2] Partners should be treated according to state laws. Patients diagnosed with chlamydia should be tested for HIV, gonorrhea, and syphilis.[2] Test of cure is not recommended for the general population. Retesting is recommended, however, 3 months after treatment, for evaluation of reinfection.

Neisseria gonorrhoeae

Gonorrhea is the second most reported STI in the United States.[1] Treatment of gonorrhea has changed over the years due to antimicrobial resistance.[3] In 2007, the CDC removed fluoroquinolones from the treatment recommendations due to resistance.[4] This leaves cephalosporins as the recommended treatment in the United States.

Currently, dual treatment with ceftriaxone and azithromycin is recommended because the use of 2 antimicrobials with different mechanisms of action may slow the emergence of resistance (**Table 2**).[2]

Patients with IgE-mediated penicillin allergy should be referred to an infectious disease specialist for management.[2]

Complicated infections
Disseminated gonococcal infection Symptoms of disseminated gonococcal infection include arthritis, tenosynovitis, and papular or pustular rash.[5] Disseminated infection can be complicated by perihepatitis, endocarditis, or meningitis. Patients with

Table 1	
Antimicrobial treatment of *Chlamydia trachomatis*	
Recommended Treatment	
Azithromycin	1 g orally single-dose observed therapy
OR	
Doxycycline	100 mg orally twice daily for 7 d
Alternative therapies	
Erythromycin	500 mg orally 4 times daily for 7 d
Erythromycin ethylsuccinate	800 mg orally 4 times daily for 7 d
Levofloxacin	500 mg orally once daily for 7 d
Ofloxacin	300 mg orally twice daily for 7 d

Data from Report MW. Annual Report 2015, National STD/AIDS Control Programme Sri Lanka. Vol 64.; 2015.

Table 2
Antimicrobial treatment of uncomplicated *Neisseria gonorrhea* infections of the cervix, urethra, rectum, and pharynx

Ceftriaxone	250 mg IM single-dose therapy
PLUS	
Azithromycin	1 g orally single-dose observed therapy

Data from Report MW. Annual Report 2015, National STD/AIDS Control Programme Sri Lanka. Vol 64.; 2015.

previously noted systemic symptoms should be referred to an infectious disease specialist for treatment.[2] Hospitalization typically is required.

Conjunctivitis Gonococcal conjunctivitis is an ocular infection caused by *Neisseria gonorrhea*, a gram-negative diplococci bacterium.[6] This infection may be spread to the eye by contact with genital secretions from a person who has a genital gonorrheal infection. Most cases occur in neonates or sexually active adults and are transmitted by contact with infected urine or genital secretions.[6] On examination, patients may have unilateral or bilateral purulent ocular discharge, conjunctival injection, chemosis, and eyelid edema.[7] The CDC recommends treatment with ceftriaxone, 250 mg intramuscularly (IM), in adults with uncomplicated infection.[6] Adjuvant treatment can include saline lavage and topical chloramphenicol or ofloxacin. In addition, patients should be treated presumptively for concurrent *Chlamydia trachomatis* infection with either azithromycin, 1 g orally, as a single dose, or doxycycline, 100 mg orally, twice daily for 7 days.[6,7]

Epididymitis Gonorrhea and chlamydia are the most common sexually transmitted bacterial infections found in sexually active men less than 35 years old who present with epididymitis. Data support the use of ceftriaxone in the treatment of epididymitis. There are no data, however, to support the use of azithromycin as a second agent. The CDC recommends doxycycline as the second agent of choice for acute epididymitis.[2] Men who engage in insertive anal sex should be treated with antimicrobials with enteric coverage, such as levofloxacin or ofloxacin, in place of doxycycline (**Tables 3** and **4**).[2]

Patient counseling and follow-up
Patients should be counseled to abstain from sexual activity for 7 days, until all partners have been treated and until symptoms, if present, have resolved.[2] A test of cure is not recommended for the general population.[2] Because drug resistance is on the rise, however, it is imperative that patients are instructed to return if symptoms persist. These patients should be evaluated for drug resistance versus reinfection. If a patient is suspected of having a cephalosporin treatment failure, a culture and antimicrobial susceptibility testing of the clinical specimens should be performed. In addition,

Table 3
Treatment of acute epididymitis

Ceftriaxone	250 mg IM single-dose therapy
PLUS	
Doxycycline	100 mg orally twice daily for 10 d

Data from Report MW. Annual Report 2015, National STD/AIDS Control Programme Sri Lanka. Vol 64.; 2015.

Table 4
Treatment of acute epididymitis in men who practice insertive anal sex

Ceftriaxone	250 mg IM single-dose therapy
PLUS	
Levofloxacin	500 mg orally once daily for 10 d
OR	
Ofloxacin	300 mg orally twice a day for 10 d

Data from Report MW. Annual Report 2015, National STD/AIDS Control Programme Sri Lanka. Vol 64.; 2015.

patients should be referred to an infectious disease specialist and the clinician should report the case to the CDC.[2]

Syphilis

Syphilis is caused by the bacteria *Treponema pallidum.*[8] It is transmitted through sexual contact and physical contact with the syphilis chancre.[8,9] Transmission also may occur through bodily fluids from bacteremia caused by syphilis.[8] Vertical transmission can occur in utero as well.[9] Syphilis is staged as primary, secondary, latent, and tertiary (**Table 5**).

Desensitization is recommended if a patient has a penicillin allergy.[2] Alternative treatments are doxycycline, ceftriaxone, penicillin G procaine, or azithromycin if a patient is unable to take penicillin G benzathine.[2,8] Doxycycline is recommended as an alternative treatment due to better dosing schedule and effectiveness than the others.[2]

Abstinence, when a chancre is present, is recommended to prevent spread of syphilis. Condoms can protect against syphilis, however, only if the chancre is completely covered.[9] Sex partners of the patient should be treated if they have had sexual contact within 90 days prior to symptom onset regardless of serologic results.[8] If sexual contact happened greater than 90 days, serologic testing can be performed and partners can be treated based on those results.[2,8] Providers can contact the local health department for help contacting partners.

Individuals who test positive for syphilis should be tested for human immunodeficiency virus (HIV) because the 2 commonly occur together.[2,8] Additionally, HIV infection has been shown to increase the likelihood of syphilis infection.[9]

Patients should be counseled on the possibility of developing a systemic reaction manifesting as fever, chills, headache, myalgias, and intensification of skin rashes (the Jarisch-Herxheimer reaction) after treatment of syphilis.[2–6] The Jarisch-Herxheimer reaction is believed to be caused by the release of endotoxin-like substances when large numbers of *Treponema pallidum* are killed by antibiotics.[2–6] This can occur during the first 24 hours of treatment in primary and secondary disease.[6]

Table 5
Treatment of syphilis

Penicillin G benzathine	2.4 million U given IM as a single dose
Alternative treatment of syphilis	
Doxycycline	100 mg given orally twice daily for 14 d

Adapted from O'Byrne P, Macpherson P. Syphilis. *BMJ.* 2019;365(June):1-11; with permission.

Titers should be checked at 6 months, 12 months, 18 months, and 24 months post-infection to ensure they are trending down.[2] A referral to an infectious disease specialist may be necessary if titers do not decline appropriately or if neurologic symptoms appear.[2]

Chancroid

Chancroid is a rare STI in the United States and is caused by a highly infectious bacterium, *Haemophilus ducreyi*.[2] There is limited diagnosis of *H ducreyi* because few laboratories have the capability of proper microbiologic diagnosis. Unlike genital herpes that often presents with initial vesicular lesions, chancroid usually presents after a 3-day to 10-day incubation with painful, purulent, and sometimes unilateral genital ulcers.[2,10] Scarring can occur in advanced cases despite treatment success. Macrolides, cephalosporin, and quinolones have been used successfully in treating chancroid for several years without any significant evidence of the emergence of resistance (**Table 6**).

Patient education should stress the use of condoms and emphasize abstinence from sex until the lesion has dried and resolved. Sex partners of the patient should be treated if they have had sexual contact within the 10 days of symptom presentation. Exposed partners should be given the same treatment as infected partners irrespective of whether or not they have symptoms. A single-dose regimen is recommended whenever possible.[1,11,12]

PARASITIC INFECTIONS
Pediculosis Pubis (Pubic Lice)

Patients with pediculosis pubis present with visible nits or lice in genital area.[11] The overwhelming symptom patient experience is itching.[11] Treatment of pediculosis pubis is with topical therapies. Visible nits should be removed and medication should be applied to all affected areas (**Table 7**).[13]

Ivermectin should be taken with food, which increases bioavailability and penetration of the drug into the epidermis.[2] Patients should be instructed to wash all clothes and bedding in hot water and dried on high heat.

Trichomonas vaginalis

Trichomonas vaginalis is caused by infection with a protozoan parasite.[1,2] Currently, nitroimidazoles are the gold standard for treatment of infection with *T vaginalis* and the only class of antimicrobials that are effective.[2] There are 2 Food and Drug Administration–approved medications in the United States, metronidazole and tinidazole. See **Table 8** for dosing recommendations. Newer evidence has shown that a 7-

Table 6 Treatment recommendations for chancroid	
Azithromycin	1 g orally as a single dose
OR	
Erythromycin	500 mg orally 3 times daily for 7 d
OR	
Ceftriaxone	250 mg IM as a single dose
OR	
Ciprofloxacin	500 mg orally twice daily for 3 d

Data from Refs.[1,10,11]

Table 7
Treatment of pediculosis pubis

Recommended treatment of pediculosis pubis	
Permethrin 1% cream rinse	Apply to affected areas and wash off after 10 min
OR	
Pyrethrins with piperonyl butoxide	Apply to affected areas and wash off after 10 min
Alternative treatment of pediculosis pubis	
Malathion 0.5% lotion	Apply to affected areas and wash off after 8–12 h
OR	
Ivermectin	250 μg/kg orally, repeat dose in 2 wk

Data from Report MW. Annual Report 2015, National STD/AIDS Control Programme Sri Lanka. Vol 64.; 2015.

day regimen of oral metronidazole may be 50% more effective at eradicating *T vaginalis* than single-dose therapy; thus, single-dose therapy should be reserved for when there is concern for medication adherence but should not be the recommendation for all patients.[14] Tinidazole has a longer half-life and fewer gastrointestinal side effects than metronidazole, although it tends to be more expensive.

Patient education should include the risk of a disulfiram-like drug reaction, including nausea, vomiting, flushing, dizziness, and headache when alcohol is consumed while taking nitroimidazoles. Patients should be advised to abstain from alcohol while taking metronidazole and tinidazole.[2] Patients also need to abstain from alcohol for at least 24 hours after completion of metronidazole and 72 hours after completion of tinidazole.[2] Patients should abstain from sex until both patient and partner have completed treatment and symptoms have resolved.[2] There is a high rate of reinfection with *T vaginalis* (17%) within 3 months of treatment among women. Therefore, the CDC recommends retesting within 3 months of treatment, regardless of treatment status of the partner.[2]

VIRAL INFECTIONS
Genital Herpes Simplex Virus

Genital herpes is caused by the herpes simplex virus (HSV). HSV is lifelong and recurrent with exacerbations and remissions.[15] There are 2 subtypes, HSV-1 and HSV-2.

Table 8
Population-specific antimicrobial treatment of *Trichomonas vaginalis*

Population	Treatment
Otherwise healthy men and women	• Metronidazole, 2 g orally in a single dose OR • Tinidazole, 2 g orally in a single dose
HIV infected women	Metronidazole, 500 mg orally twice daily for 7 d
Pregnant women	Metronidazole, 2 g orally in a single dose
Treatment failure	Metronidazole, 500 mg orally twice daily for 7 d
Nitroimidazole resistance	Metronidazole or tinidazole, 2 g daily for 7 d
IgE-mediated allergy	Desensitization to nitroimidazoles with an allergy specialist

Data from Report MW. Annual Report 2015, National STD/AIDS Control Programme Sri Lanka. Vol 64.; 2015.

Classically, HSV-2 caused genital herpes and HSV-1 caused oral lesions but cross-over is common.[15] Patients often are asymptomatic. Symptomatic patients may experience painful blisters or sores.[15] Transmission occurs through contact with an active herpes lesion to mucosa, saliva, or genital fluid.[15,16] It also can occur when patients do not have an active herpes lesion and the virus sheds. Asymptomatic genital viral shedding is the most common type of transmission.[17]

Treatment approach (episodic vs suppressive)

Treatment of HSV can be either episodic or suppressive. Episodic therapy is aimed to treat the acute, painful lesions,[17] whereas suppressive therapy is aimed at decreasing lesion occurrences.[17] Additionally, suppressive therapy decreases overall HSV viral shedding.[17] Suppressive therapy has been shown to decrease HSV outbreaks up to 80%.[2] Initiating treatment can decrease symptom duration significantly (**Tables 9 and 10**).[16]

First-line treatment of initial HSV infection is with acyclovir, valacyclovir, or famciclovir.[17] After the initial lesion outbreak, dosing changes slightly to suppressive dosing. See **Table 11** for suppressive treatment options. Patient adherence is better with once-a-day dosing. Therefore, valacyclovir is used more frequently.[17] Episodic dosing is recommended for recurrent outbreaks of genital lesions and should be started within 24 hours of prodromal symptoms.[2] Episodic treatment also can be with famciclovir, acyclovir, or valacyclovir. Famciclovir dosing is preferred because it is twice a day for 1 day.[2] Supportive therapies include sitz baths for comfort and analgesics for pain.[17]

Patient counseling and follow-up

Patients should be made aware that although HSV infection is lifelong, it is manageable with treatment.[17] Medication adherence is important for those who are on suppressive therapy to prevent outbreaks.[2] Patients with HSV can remain sexually active but should be advised to discuss their status with sexual partners.[17] Abstinence is encouraged during episodic outbreaks.[2,17] Condoms can help decrease transmission to vulnerable partners but are more effective in infected men with noninfected women.[17] Condoms are not as effective in infected women with noninfected male partners.[17]

Patients are concerned about the long-term implications of HSV. There is patient-reported depression, anxiety, shame, anger, and fear associated with HSV diagnosis; thus, mental health should be addressed.[2,17] With appropriate medical and mental health interventions, this condition can be controlled adequately. Counseling both patient and partner can be equally benefical.[15]

Partners of those with HSV need to have serologic testing and education.[17] Partners may be asymptomatic and not know their HSV status.[2] If serologic testing is positive,

Table 9	
Herpes simplex virus initial treatment	
Acyclovir	400 mg orally 2 times daily for 7–10 d
OR	
Valacyclovir (preferred due to convenience)	1 g orally twice daily for 7–10 d
OR	
Famciclovir	250 mg orally three times daily for 7–10 d

Data from Report MW. *Annual Report 2015, National STD/AIDS Control Programme Sri Lanka.* Vol 64.; 2015. And Gnann JW, Whitley RJ. Genital herpes. *N Engl J Med.* 2016;375(7):666-674.

Table 10 Herpes simplex virus suppressive treatment	
Acyclovir	400 mg orally twice daily
OR	
Valacyclovir	500 mg orally once daily
OR	
Famciclovir	250 mg orally twice daily

Data from Report MW. Annual Report 2015, National STD/AIDS Control Programme Sri Lanka. Vol 64.; 2015.

episodic or suppressive therapy should be recommended as for any HSV patient.[2] The continued need for suppressive therapy should be evaluated at each follow-up visit.[2]

Hepatitis B

Hepatitis B virus (HBV) infection is the most common chronic viral infection in the world, affecting more than 350 million people worldwide, making it a major public health problem.[1,2] There are 3 major modes of transmission of HBV: contact with blood or semen, perinatal transmission from infected mothers to neonates, and lastly unsafe injections, blood transfusions, or dialysis. The manifestations of HBV varies both in acute and chronic situations. HBV infection can be self-limited or chronic.[18,19]

Treatment

Treatment of HBV infection mostly is supportive because no specific therapy is available for persons with acute hepatitis B.[20] Referral to a specialist is indicated for persons with chronic HBV infection.

Prevention

HBV infection can be prevented by avoiding transmission from infected people and by inducing immunity in unexposed people.[20,21] To decrease the global burden of HBV infection, the following are important steps in the prevention of HBV transmission: screening of blood donors for hepatitis B surface antigen (HBsAg) and implementation of universal precautions, counseling infected people to prevent transmission, screening, and vaccination of at-risk adults and universal vaccination of neonates.[21] See **Box 1** for indications for hepatitis B vaccine.

The introduction to hepatitis B vaccine has led to a decrease in the incidence of the infection. The following 2 products have been approved for the prevention of HBV infection: hepatitis B immune globulin for postexposure prophylaxis and hepatitis B vaccine. Pre-exposure vaccination is the best way to prevent hepatitis B infection.[20]

On the other hand, hepatitis B vaccine provides protection when used for both pre-exposure vaccination and postexposure prophylaxis. There are 2 available monovalent hepatitis B vaccines for use in the United States—Recombivax HB (Merk & Co., INC., United States) and Engerix-B (GlaxoSmithKline, United States). Twinrix

Table 11 Herpes simplex virus episodic treatment	
Famciclovir	1 g orally twice daily for 1 d

Data from Report MW. Annual Report 2015, National STD/AIDS Control Programme Sri Lanka. Vol 64.; 2015.

Box 1
Indications for vaccination against hepatitis B virus infection[18,21]

All infants

All children and adolescents not previously vaccinated

High-risk adults
- MSM
- People who have multiple sexual partners
- Injection drug users
- Patients in institutions
- Patients on hemodialysis
- Health care workers and public safety workers
- Spouses, sexual partners, or household members of people who carry HBV

Reprinted with permission from Elsevier. Cassisi JA. Hepatitis B vaccine. Prim Care Update Ob Gyns. 1999;6(6):209-11; with permission. And Trépo C, Chan HLY, Lok A. Hepatitis B virus infection. Lancet. 2014;384(9959):2053-63.

(GlaxoSmithKline Biologicals., United States), a combination of hepatitis A and hepatitis B vaccine, is available for use in persons age 18 and older.[20] The recommended hepatitis B vaccine dose and schedule vary by product and age of recipient. Generally well tolerated, the vaccine can be administered simultaneously with other vaccines and should be administered in the deltoid muscle. Hepatitis B vaccine is recommended for all unvaccinated persons at risk for HBV infection; see **Box 1**.

Education Persons with HBsAG should be advised to avoid or limit alcohol consumption because of the effects on the liver.[18,20,21] They also should check with their health care provider before taking any new or over-the-counter medications. They should refrain from donating blood or blood products, body organs, tissue, or semen as well as refrain from sharing household articles that could be contaminated with blood.[18,20]

Hepatitis C

Hepatitis C virus (HCV) is the most common chronic blood-borne infection in the United States.[2] HCV is the leading cause of liver-related morbidity and mortality worldwide.[22] Although not transmitted efficiently through sex, sexual transmission can occur, especially among persons with HIV infection and among men who have sex with men (MSM).[20] Primary mode of transmission is through shared needles and paraphernalia. Newly infected persons may be unaware of the infection because they are asymptomatic or have mild illness. Occupational and perinatal exposure can result in HCV transmission.[20]

Screening for HCV is recommended for the following persons: individuals born between 1945 to 1965 and persons with a recognized exposure or at high risk for infection (those with past or current injection use, with long-term hemodialysis, with intranasal drug use, with an unregulated tattoo, or being born to a mother with HCV infection). Acute HCV is a reportable condition in the United States.[23]

Treatment
Care of a patient with HCV infection requires consultation specialists knowledgeable about management of HCV infection. Hepatitis A and B vaccination should be administered if the patient is eligible.

Treatment of chronic HCV is based on guidelines from the Infectious Diseases Society of America and the American Association for the Study of Liver Diseases, in collaboration with the International Antiviral Society–USA.[24,25] They recommend treatment decisions be based on individual patient disease state and associated comorbidity. See **Table 12** for medication options.

Management of sex partners with hepatitis C virus

Heterosexuals and MSM with HCV infection who have more than 1 partner, especially those with concurrent HIV infection, should use male latex condoms to protect their partners against HIV and HCV acquisition.[2] Partners of persons with HCV and HIV infection should be tested for HCV and HIV if their status is not known. Heterosexual couples in a long-term monogamous relationship should discuss the need for testing with their partners but do not need to change their sexual practices.[20]

Prevention of hepatitis C

There is no available vaccine for hepatitis C. Immune globulin prophylaxis is not effective in HCV infection prevention after exposure.[20] Immediate identification of acute HCV infection, however, is needed for better outcome. Primary and secondary prevention strategies are required to reduce the burden of HCV infection in the United States.[20]

Patient education

Persons with HCV should be instructed against alcohol consumption and taking medicines that have not been approved by their clinician because some of them may be hepatotoxic.[2] They should be advised not to donate blood, tissue, organs or semen; not to share items that might have blood; and to cover cuts and sores to avoid transmission to others. Injection drug users should be encouraged to participate in substance abuse treatment program, including relapse prevention.[23,26,27] Persons who are not yet immune to hepatitis A and be should be encouraged to get vaccinated.

Human Papillomavirus Infection

Human papillomavirus (HPV) is the most common STI, especially in those in the late teens and early 20s.[20] HPV infections mostly are asymptomatic, unrecognized, and self-limited. Mode of transmission is by skin-to-skin contact via vaginal, anal, or oral sex routes with someone who has the virus. Approximately 100 types of HPV have been identified and at least 40 of them can affect the genital area. HPV types 16 and 18 are high-risk, oncogenic HPV infections that cause most cervical, penile, vaginal, vulvar, and oropharyngeal cancers and precancers. HPV types 6 and 11 are low-risk and nononcogenic and cause genital warts and recurrent respiratory papillomatosis.[20]

Table 12 Treatment of hepatitis C	
Epclusa (sofosbuvir-velpatasvir)	400 mg/100 mg orally daily Take for 12 wk regardless of cirrhosis status.
Mavyret (glecaprevir-pibrentasvir)	100 mg/40 mg, 3 tablets orally daily Take for 8 wk if no cirrhosis, or 12 wk if cirrhosis is present. Can be given to patients 12 y and older.
Harvoni (ledipasvir-sofosbuvir)	90 mg/400 mg orally daily Take for 8 wk if no cirrhosis, or 12 wk if cirrhosis is present. Approved for patients 12 y of age and older.

Human papillomavirus prevention

Sexual abstinence and HPV vaccines are primary prevention mechanisms against the infection.[20] Abstaining from sexual activity, however, is the most reliable method of preventing genital HPV infection. Limiting the number of sexual partners as well as consistent and correct condom use can help decrease an individual's chances of infection (**Table 13**).[20]

HPV vaccines can be administered regardless of history of anogenital warts, abnormal Papanicolaou/HPV tests, or anogenital precancer. Vaccination is not associated with initiation of sexual activity or sexual risk behaviors or perceptions about STIs.[20] HPV vaccines are not recommended for use in pregnant women.

Treatment

Individuals with HPV do not seek treatment because they usually are asymptomatic. There is no medical indication to treat an asymptomatic wart that was discovered incidentally on physical examination.[2] The main indication for treatment of vulvovaginal warts is removal of the wart and alleviation of bothersome symptoms, such as pruritus, vaginal discharge, pain, dyspareunia, and so forth, or psychological distress.[1,10] There is no treatment of the virus; there are treatments for the health problems that HPV can cause.[20] Treatment of anogenital warts should be guided by wart size, number, and anatomic site; patient preference; cost of treatment; convenience; adverse effects; and provider preference. Medical treatment of HPV can be administered at home or in a health care provider's office (**Table 14**). There are 2 treatment modalities for HPV infection—those that directly destroy the wart (cytodestructive therapies) and those that work through patients' immune system to clear the wart (immune-mediated therapies).[24] Some clinicians employ combination therapy because all available treatments have shortcomings. Follow-up visits after several weeks of therapy are indicated for providers to assess response to treatment.

Follow-up and counseling

Anogenital warts respond within 3 months of therapy. Immunosuppression and treatment compliance are factors that might affect response to therapy. Genital warts may go away without treatment. Women with genital warts do not need Papanicolaou tests more than other women. Some persons may experience psychosocial challenges after the diagnosis requiring mental health evaluation.[2] Treatment of genital warts does not cure the virus. HPV might remain present and can be transmitted to partners after the warts are gone. Use of condoms might lower the chances of transmission.[2]

Management of sex partners

Current sexual partners should be notified of the infection because the type of HPV that causes warts can be transmitted.[2] HPV testing of sex partners is not recommended.

Table 13		
Human papillomavirus vaccines approved for clinical use		
Gardasil	Quadrivalent HPV vaccine	Targets HPV types 6, 11, 16, and 18
Gardasil 9	9-valent vaccine[a]	Targets HPV types 6, 11, 16, 18, 31, 33, 45, 52, and 58
Cervarix	Bivalent vaccine	Targets HPV types 16 and 18

[a] Only vaccine available in the United States.

From Parameshwaran V, Cockbain BC, Hillyard M, Price JR. Is the Lack of Specific Lesbian, Gay, Bisexual, Transgender and Queer/Questioning (LGBTQ) Health Care Education in Medical School a Cause for Concern? Evidence From a Survey of Knowledge and Practice Among UK Medical Students. *J Homosex.* 2017;64(3):367-381; with permission.

Table 14
Recommended regimens for external anogenital warts (ie, penis, groin, scrotum, vulva, perineum, external anus, and perianus)

Patient applied	
Imiquimod, 3.75% or 5% cream	Apply once at bedtime 3 times 1 wk for up to 16 wk. Wash with soap and water hours after application. Avoid during pregnancy.
OR	
Podofilox, 0.5% solution or gel	Using finger, apply to anogenital warts twice a day followed by no therapy for 4 d. Can be repeated for up to 4 cycles. Podofilox is contraindicated in pregnancy.
OR	
Sinecatechins, 15% ointment	Apply using finger 3 times daily. This product should not be continued after 16 wk. Do not use during pregnancy
Provider administered	
Cryotherapy with liquid nitrogen or cryoprobe	Health provider must be trained on the proper use of this therapy to avoid overtreatment and under treatment. Pain and blistering are common.
OR	
Surgical removal either by tangential scissor excision, tangential shave excision, curettage, laser, or electrosurgery	Surgical removal requires clinical training, additional equipment, and longer office visit.
OR	
TCA or BCA 80%–90%	TCA/BCA should be applied only to warts. TCA/BCA can be repeated weekly in needed

Abbreviations: BCA, bichloroacetic acid; TCA, trichloroacetic acid.
From Parameshwaran V, Cockbain BC, Hillyard M, Price JR. Is the Lack of Specific Lesbian, Gay, Bisexual, Transgender and Queer/Questioning (LGBTQ) Health Care Education in Medical School a Cause for Concern? Evidence From a Survey of Knowledge and Practice Among UK Medical Students. *J Homosex.* 2017;64(3):367-381; with permission.

Special considerations

High-grade squamous intraepithelial lesions An atypical wart might reveal high-grade squamous intraepithelial lesion or cancer of the anogenital tract after biopsy.[2] Referral to a specialist for treatment is recommended.

Cervical cancer—human papillomavirus tests for cervical cancer screening Cervical cancer is the only HPV-associated cancer for which routine screening is recommended. Major medical organizations like the American College of Surgeons, American College of Obstetricians and Gynecologists (ACOG), and the US Preventive Services Task Force recommend that cervical screening should be performed starting at the age of 21 and continue through the age 65 to prevent invasive cervical cancer.[2] Annual cervical cancer screening no longer is recommended for all women. Papanicolaou testing is recommended every 3 years from ages 21 through 29 years. During age 30 through 65 years, women should either receive a Papanicolaou test every 3 years or a Papanicolaou test plus HPV test (cotest) every 5 years.[2] The Papanicolaou test is not a screening test for STIs. All women, however, should receive cervical cancer screening regardless of their sexual orientation.

Human Immunodeficiency Virus

HIV affects the CD4 cells, which are part of the immune system that help to fight infections.[28] CD4 cells are also called T lymphocytes or T cells. Over time, the virus decreases overall CD4 cell count, leading to worsening of the HIV infection.[28] The later, more serious stage of HIV is acquired immunodeficiency syndrome. CD4 numbers are monitored by health care providers to determine severity of illness.[28] It is transmitted from body fluids, such as blood, rectal fluids, vaginal fluids, semen, and breastmilk.[28] In order for transmission to occur, these fluids then have to contact a mucous membrane.[28]

Treatment approach

HIV is complex and requires treatment with a combination of medications generally referred to as antiretroviral therapy (ART).[29] The goal of ART in HIV is to suppress the replication of the virus, reconstitute the immune system, and slow progression of disease.[29] ART therapy also has the potential to decrease transmission to others.[29] Treatment is able to be managed only by a trained HIV care provider. There are 5 classes of medications that are Food and Drug Administration approved to treat HIV: reverse transcriptase inhibitors, protease inhibitors, fusion inhibitors, chemokine receptor 5 antagonists, and integrase strand transfer inhibitors. Reverse transcriptase inhibitors prevent reproduction of HIV.[29] The 2 types of reverse transcriptase inhibitors are non-nucleoside reverse transcriptase inhibitors and nucleoside reverse transcriptase inhibitors (NRTIs).[29] Protease inhibitors block the protease enzymes in CD4 cells, which decreased HIV production.[29] Fusion inhibitors inhibit HIV from infecting new CD4 cells.[29] Chemokine receptor 5 antagonists block the chemokine receptor 5, which then decreases HIV from infecting cells.[29] Integrase strand transfer inhibitors block the integrase enzyme that helps with HIV replication.[29]

ART should be started on any patient with HIV.[30] The goal of ART is viral suppression.[28] First-line ART treatment of adults and adolescents with HIV is with an integrase strand transfer inhibitor, dolutegravir, in combination with an NRTI backbone (2 NRTI medications).[31]

Treatment of special populations

There are some studies to suggest that transgender women have lower ART success in term of CD4 counts.[28,32] There is a concern in the transgender women community that ART will interfere with hormone therapy, which effects adherence and, therefore, decreases CD4 counts.[28] There are several ART combinations that do not have interactions with hormone therapy and requires extensive patient education.[33]

Patient counseling

Medication adherence for ART is burdensome because it is a lifelong regimen. There also are risk factors for nonadherence: adverse drug reactions, health literacy, stigma of the condition, and socioeconomic status.[29] There are many potential side effects and adverse drug reactions to ART medications. Gastrointestinal symptoms, such as nausea, vomiting, and diarrhea, and headache, are the most frequent adverse drug reactions that can have an impact on adherence.[34,35] These reactions usually are short lasting.

Abstinence could help decrease the spread of HIV. The PARTNER (Partners of People on ART - A New Evaluation of the Risks) study noted that condoms may reduce transmission to sexual partners and, therefore, should be recommended by health care providers.[36]

Partners of those who have HIV need to be screened routinely to ensure transmission has not occurred. Historically, treatment of sexual partner is not done routinely unless HIV testing was positive. Oral pre-exposure prophylaxis (PrEP) now is available to those at substantial risk for acquiring HIV.[30] In the United States, there are 2 approved forms of PrEP. Truvada is prescribed in a 1-pill combination of emtricitabine (FTC) and tenofovir disoproxil fumarate.[31] Descovy is prescribed in a 1-pill combination of emtricitabine (FTC) and tenofovir alafenamide. Other forms of PrEP are being investigated to bring down cost and improved medication adherence.[37] HIV and renal function testing are performed regularly while patients are on PrEP.[30] PrEP offers emotional benefits for partners as well: improved partner relationships, decreased anxiety, and decreased HIV stigma.[38]

Those who are exposed to HIV that are not on PrEP need postexposure prophylaxis, preferably 72 hours after exposure.[30] Treatment includes tenofovir disoproxil fumarate and lamivudine (3TC) as treatment backbone plus lopinavir or atazanavir with low-dose ritonavir as a third medication.[30] Treatment usually is prescribed for 28 days.[30]

Due to the chronicity of HIV, mental health conditions are common and are essential to treat.[39] Depression is the condition seen to coincide the most with HIV.[39] Anxiety, substance abuse, and stress are seen as well in patients living with HIV.[29,40] These psychological conditions need a mixed modality treatment plan, including a combination of cognitive behavioral therapy, medication, meditation, and stress management.[40] Additionally, mental disorders can lead to medication adherence issues.

Follow-up

HIV and PrEP patients need to be under the care of trained providers. CD4 counts are checked routinely with those who have HIV to ensure that treatment is effective.[41] Patients may need behavioral health, mental health, or substance abuse referrals related to diagnosis.[41]

SUMMARY

STI rates have increased overall from 2017 to 2018 with profound implications for public health.[1] Primary care providers need to be aware of available pharmacologic therapies. Primary care providers also need to be mindful of populations who may need altered STI treatment, including those who are pregnancy, those who have HIV-positive status, MSM, and those with mental health conditions. Patients should be counseled on methods of disease transmission and preventive measures to prevent spread to sexual partners.

Antimicrobial therapy for bacterial STIs must be selected carefully to eradicate disease and to prevent antimicrobial resistance. Although there is no cure for most of the viral STIs, medications and precautions may help reduce disease transmission. It is imperative that primary care providers are up to date on current pharmacologic recommendations in the treatment of STIs. Appropriate treatment minimizes negative health related outcomes and aids in the reduction of the STI global burden.

DISCLOSURE

The authors have nothing to disclose.

REFERENCES

1. HHS, CDC, Oid, NCHHSTP, DSTDP. Sexually Transmitted Disease Surveillance 2018. 2018. Available at: https://www.cdc.gov/std/stats18/STDSurveillance2018-full-report.pdf.

2. Report MW. Annual Report 2015, National STD/AIDS Control Programme Sri Lanka. Vol 64.; 2015. Available at: https://www.cdc.gov/mmwr/preview/mmwrhtml/rr6403a1.htm?s_cid=rr6403a1_w.

3. Workowski KA, Berman SM, Douglas JM. Emerging antimicrobial resistance in Neisseria gonorrhoeae: Urgent need to strengthen prevention strategies (Annals of Internal Medicine (2008) 148, (606-613)). Ann Intern Med 2008;148(11):888.

4. CDC. Update to CDC's Sexually Transmitted Diseases Treatment Guidelines, 2006: Fluoroquinolones No Longer Recommended for Treatment of Gonococcal Infections. 2007. Available at: https://www.cdc.gov/mmwr/preview/mmwrhtml/mm5614a3.htm. Accessed October 22, 2019.

5. Belkacem A, Caumes E, Ouanich J, et al. Changing patterns of disseminated gonococcal infection in france: Cross-sectional data 2009-2011. Sex Transm Infect 2013;89(8):613-5.

6. del Rio C, Hall G, Holmes K, et al. Update to CDC's sexually transmitted diseases treatment guidelines, 2010: Oral cephalosporins no longer a recommended treatment for gonococcal infections. Morb Mortal Wkly Rep 2012;61(31):590-4.

7. Haimovici R, Roussel TJ. Treatment of gonococcal conjunctivitis with single-dose intramuscular ceftriaxone. Am J Ophthalmol 1989;107(5):511-4.

8. O'Byrne P, Macpherson P. Syphilis. BMJ 2019;365:1-11.

9. Stoltey JE, Cohen SE. Syphilis transmission: a review of the current evidence. Sex Health 2015;12(2):103-9.

10. Lewis DA, Mitjà O. Haemophilus ducreyi: From sexually transmitted infection to skin ulcer pathogen. Curr Opin Infect Dis 2016;29(1):52-7.

11. Organization WH. W O R L D H E a Lt H O R G a N I Z At I O N W O R L D H E a Lt H O R G a N I Z At I O N Guidelines for the Management of Sexually Transmitted Infections Wo R Ld Health O R G an I Zati O N W O R L D H E a Lt H O R G a N I Z At I O N W O R L D H E a Lt H O. 2001. Available at: http://www.who.int/HIV_AIDS/. Accessed October 22, 2019.

12. Wiley DJ, Douglas J, Beutner K, et al. External genital warts: diagnosis, treatment, and prevention. Clin Infect Dis 2002;35(s2):S210-24.

13. Salavastru CM, Chosidow O, Janier M, et al. European guideline for the management of pediculosis pubis. J Eur Acad Dermatol Venereol 2017;31(9):1425-8.

14. Kissinger P, Adamski A. Trichomoniasis and HIV interactions: A review. Sex Transm Infect 2013;89(6):426-33.

15. McQuillan G, Kruszon-Moran D, Flagg EW, et al. Prevalence of Herpes Simplex Virus Type 1 and Type 2 in Persons Aged 14-49: United States, 2015-2016. NCHS Data Brief 2018;(304):1-8.

16. Ng BE, Rutherford GW, White AB, et al. Antiviral therapy for genital herpes for prevention of HIV transmission. Cochrane Database Syst Rev 2018;2018(5). https://doi.org/10.1002/14651858.CD006492.pub3.

17. Gnann JW, Whitley RJ. Genital herpes. N Engl J Med 2016;375(7):666-74.

18. Cassisi JA. Hepatitis B vaccine. Prim Care Update Ob Gyns 1999;6(6):209-11.

19. Guidelines for the Prevention, Care and Treatment of Persons with Chronic Hepatitis B Infection. Geneva: World Health Organization; 2015. Available at: https://apps.who.int/iris/bitstream/handle/10665/154590/9789241549059_eng.pdf?sequence=1.

20. Parameshwaran V, Cockbain BC, Hillyard M, et al. Is the lack of specific lesbian, gay, bisexual, transgender and queer/questioning (LGBTQ) health care education in medical school a cause for concern? evidence from a survey of knowledge and practice among UK medical students. J Homosex 2017;64(3):367-81.

21. Trépo C, Chan HLY, Lok A. Hepatitis B virus infection. Lancet 2014;384(9959): 2053–63.
22. Razavi H, Robbins S, Zeuzem S, et al. Hepatitis C virus prevalence and level of intervention required to achieve the WHO targets for elimination in the European Union by 2030: a modelling study. Lancet Gastroenterol Hepatol 2017;2(5): 325–36.
23. Zibbell JE, Asher AK, Patel RC, et al. Increases in acute hepatitis C virus infection related to a growing opioid epidemic and associated injection drug use, United States, 2004 to 2014. Am J Public Health 2018;108(2):175–81.
24. No WV. Errata to FDA Licensure of Bivalent Human Papillomavirus Vaccine (HPV2, Cervarix) for Use in Females and Updated HPV Vaccination Recommendations from the Advisory Committee on Immunization Practices (ACIP). Morb Mortal Wkly Rep 2010;59(36):1184.
25. Sidharthan S, Kohli A, Sims Z, et al. Utility of hepatitis c viral load monitoring on Direct-Acting antiviral therapy. Clin Infect Dis 2015;60(12):1743–51.
26. Kim WR. The burden of hepatitis C in the United States. Hepatology 2002;36(5 l):30–4.
27. Zibbell JE, Iqbal K, Patel RC, et al. Increases in hepatitis C virus infection related to injection drug use among persons aged ≤30 years — Kentucky, Tennessee, Virginia, and West Virginia, 2006–2012. Morb Mortal Wkly Rep 2015;64(17): 453–8.
28. HIV: Basic statistics. Centers for Disease Control and Prevention. 2019. Available at: https://www.cdc.gov/hiv/basics/statistics.html. Accessed October 16, 2019.
29. Bhatti AB, Usman M, Kandi V. Current scenario of HIV/AIDS, treatment options, and major challenges with compliance to antiretroviral therapy. Cureus 2016; 8(3):1–12.
30. World Health Organization. Guideline on When To Start Antiretroviral Therapy and on Pre-Exposure Prophylaxis for HIV. 2015;(September):1-76. Available at: https://apps.who.int/iris/bitstream/handle/10665/186275/9789241509565_eng.pdf;jsessionid=DDB0089A3EC1139F1AF1262202B89C2D?sequence=1.
31. Update of recommendations on first- and second-line antiretroviral regimens. Geneva, Switzerland: World Health Organization; 2019 (WHO/CDS/HIV/19.15). License: CC BY-NC-SA 3.0 IGO. Available at: https://apps.who.int/iris/bitstream/handle/10665/325892/WHO-CDS-HIV-19.15-eng.pdf?ua=1.
32. Wiewel EW, Torian LV, Merchant P, et al. HIV diagnoses and care among transgender persons and comparison with men who have sex with men: New York City, 2006-2011. Am J Public Health 2016;106(3):497–502.
33. Panel on Antiretroviral Guidelines for Adults and Adolescents. Guidelines for the Use of Antiretroviral Agents in Adults and Adolescents with HIV. Department of Health and Human Services. Available at: http://www.aidsinfo.nih.gov/ContentFiles/AdultandAdolescentGL.pdf. Accessed July 1, 2020.
34. Tadesse WT, Mekonnen AB, Tesfaye WH, et al. Self-reported adverse drug reactions and their influence on highly active antiretroviral therapy in HIV infected patients: A cross sectional study. BMC Pharmacol Toxicol 2014;15(1).
35. Wood E, Montaner JSG, Chan K, et al. Socioeconomic status, access to triple therapy, and survival from HIV-disease since 1996. AIDS 2002;16(15):2065–72.
36. Rodger AJ, Cambiano V, Bruun T, et al. Sexual activity without condoms and risk of HIV transmission in serodifferent couples when the HIV-positive partner is using suppressive antiretroviral therapy. JAMA 2016;316(2):171–81.

37. World Health Organization. Appropriate Medicines: Options for Pre-Exposure Prophylaxis. Meeting Report. 2016;(March):1-45. Available at: https://apps.who.int/iris/handle/10665/273934. Accessed October 22, 2019.
38. Grant RM, Koester KA. What people want from sex and preexposure prophylaxis. Curr Opin HIV AIDS 2016;11(1):3–9.
39. Nanni MG, Caruso R, Mitchell AJ, et al. Depression in HIV infected patients: a review. Curr Psychiatry Rep 2014;17(1):530.
40. van Luenen S, Garnefski N, Spinhoven P, et al. The benefits of psychosocial interventions for mental health in people living with HIV: a systematic review and meta-analysis. AIDS Behav 2018;22(1):9–42.
41. Centers for Disease Control and Prevention, Health Resources and Services Administration, National Institutes of Health, American Academy of HIV Medicine, Association of Nurses in AIDS Care, International Association of Providers of AIDS Care, the National Minority AIDS Council, and Urban Coalition for HIV/AIDS Prevention Services. Recommendations for HIV Prevention with Adults and Adolescents with HIV in the United States; 2014. Available at: http://stacks.cdc.gov/view/cdc/26062.

Proctitis in Men Who Have Sex with Men

Julia M. Steed, PhD, APRN, FNP-BC*, Queen Henry-Okafor, PhD, FNP-BC, PMHNP-BC,
Courtney J. Pitts, DNP, MPH, FNP-BC

KEYWORDS

- Proctitis • Sexually transmitted infections • Men who have sex with men (MSM)
- Human immunodeficiency virus (HIV)

KEY POINTS

- The rate of sexually transmitted infections is disproportionately higher in individuals 15 to 24 years old and in men who have sex with men (MSM).
- Proctitis is an inflammatory condition caused by sexually transmitted infections that often goes misdiagnosed in MSM.
- Misdiagnosis is often due to a clinical presentation that mirrors common gastrointestinal disorders.
- Health care providers should be knowledgeable of the clinical presentation and appropriate testing to ensure accurate diagnosis and timely treatment.

Sexually transmitted infections (STIs) are diseases that are transmitted from 1 person to another person through acts of vaginal, anal, or oral intercourse. As of 2017, it was estimated that there were approximately 20 million new STI diagnoses in the United States each year.[1] More than half of these new diagnoses occur among individuals aged 15 to 24 years.[2] The 3 notifiable STIs in the United States include *Neisseria gonorrhoeae*, *Chlamydia trachomatis*, and *Treponema pallidum*. Although reported rates of STIs have increased among men and women over the 2017 to 2018 period, the most dramatic rate increase has been among men who have sex with men (MSM).[2] The higher rates may be attributed to an increased screening or transmission among this population.[2] The high rate of STIs among MSM results in the increased incidence of STI-related diagnoses, such as proctitis. Proctitis is a common, but often misdiagnosed condition experienced by MSM who present to primary care, urgent care, and emergency settings. It is important that health care providers be knowledgeable of the pathophysiology, risk factors, and clinical presentation of proctitis among MSM for accurate and timely management.

Vanderbilt University School of Nursing, 461 21st Avenue South, Nashville, TN 37240, USA
* Corresponding author.
E-mail address: julia.m.steed@vanderbilt.edu

Nurs Clin N Am 55 (2020) 325–335
https://doi.org/10.1016/j.cnur.2020.05.003   **nursing.theclinics.com**
0029-6465/20/© 2020 Elsevier Inc. All rights reserved.

BACKGROUND

Proctitis is one of 3 gastrointestinal syndromes caused by STIs.[3] It is the inflammation of the anal canal and distal rectum that can be caused by infectious or noninfectious pathogens (**Table 1**).[4] The most common infectious pathogens include *N gonorrhoeae*, *C trachomatis*, *T pallidum*, and herpes simplex virus (HSV), with *C trachomatis* and *N gonorrhoeae* being the second and third leading causes in MSM, respectively.[4–6] Individuals with proctitis may complain of anorectal pain, rectal bleeding, rectal discharge, urgency, diarrhea, incontinence, pelvic pain, or tenesmus.[3,6]

Proctocolitis and enteritis are the remaining gastrointestinal syndromes caused by STIs. An individual with proctocolitis may present clinically with symptoms similar to proctitis, but with additional complaints of diarrhea and abdominal cramps.[3] However, proctocolitis typically results in the inflammation of the colonic mucosa extending to 12 cm above the anus.[3] A clinical presentation of enteritis typically consists of complaints of diarrhea and abdominal cramping in the absence of signs of proctitis or procticolitis.[3] Unfortunately, these symptoms are nonspecific and mimic other gastrointestinal disease processes commonly seen in primary care, urgent care, and emergency settings, leading to a high rate of misdiagnosis (**Box 1**).

Other causes of proctitis include radiation therapy, inflammatory bowel disease (IBD), infections, antibiotics, diversion proctitis, food protein–induced proctitis, and eosinophilic proctitis. Radiation proctitis is inflammation and damage to the lower part of the colon secondary to ionizing radiation exposure.[7] Individuals who have had radiation therapy directed at their rectum, colon, prostate, cervix, or ovaries have an increased risk of developing radiation proctitis. Having an IBD such as Crohn disease or ulcerative colitis increases the risk of proctitis.[4] Infections associated with food-borne bacteria, such as salmonella, shigella, and campylobacter, are another cause of proctitis. Although necessary to ameliorate symptoms related to bacterium-causing infections, antibiotic use may alter the normal flora of the rectum, predisposing it to infection by other organisms.[8] Diversion proctitis may occur secondary to surgical interventions in the colon in which stool passage is diverted from the rectum.[7,9] Food protein–induced proctitis may be experienced in infants who consume either cow's milk or soy-based formula or those breast-fed by mothers who eat dairy products.[10] Eosinophilic proctitis affects children younger than 2 years old and occurs when eosinophils build up in the lining of the rectum. Although STIs are

Table 1 Infectious and noninfectious pathogens of proctitis	
Infectious	**Noninfectious**
Enteric infections • Campylobacter • Shigella • *Escherichia coli* • Salmonella • Amebiasis	• Medical radiation • Rectal instrumentation and trauma • Autoimmune disease of the colon • Side effect of medical treatments
Sexually transmitted infections • Gonorrhea • Chlamydia, syphilis • Herpes simplex virus • Lymphogranuloma venereum chancroid • Cytomegalovirus • Human papillomavirus	

Box 1
Common misdiagnoses

- Irritable bowel syndrome
- Crohn disease
- Ulcerative colitis
- "Rectal pain"
- Hemorrhoids
- Rectal cancer
- Radiation-associated proctitis/proctopathy
- Diversion colitis
- Ischemia

---

the most common cause of proctitis, it is of utter importance that health care providers take a thorough history during the clinical encounter.

SEXUALLY TRANSMITTED INFECTIONS

The presence of STIs in MSM triggers an inflammatory process within the anal mucosa, resulting in complaints of rectal symptoms.[11] Different pathogens typically infect varying sites of the anorectal canal. *N gonorrhoeae* and *C trachomatis*, also known as gonorrhea and chlamydia, infect the columnar epithelium when they occur in the rectum. Among MSM, most rectal infections caused by gonorrhea and chlamydia are asymptomatic, because the rectum itself has few sensory nerve endings, and infections sparing the anus may be painless.[12]

There are 2 strains of chlamydia:lymphogranuloma venereum (LGV) and nonlymphogranuloma venereum (non-LGV). Non-LGV strains of chlamydia are commonly identified as the cause for proctitis. Although asymptomatic in a high proportion of people, symptoms may arise 5 to 10 days after exposure and include pruritus ani, constipation, mucopurulent anal discharge, bleeding, pain, and tenesmus.[13,14] LGV infections among MSM were mostly identified in western Europe around 2005, mainly in human immunodeficiency virus (HIV)-infected patients undertaking high-risk sexual activities.[15–17] LGV infections were also found in parts of Africa, Asia, the Caribbean, and South America until around 2003.[18] Current rates of reported LGV in Europe, Asia, Africa, and the United States are likely an underestimation of the true prevalence.[19] Although this bacterium has 15 clinical serotypes, only L1, L2, and L3 are found to cause proctitis.[18] Onset of LGV includes a 3-stage clinical course: an incubation period, appearance of ulcerated papules, and lymph node necroinflammation.[18]

HSV may be acquired through both anal and oral-anal intercourse. Most infections are from HSV type 2, although HSV-1 is also common.[20] HSV-causing proctitis predominantly affects the perianal skin and anal canal, but may extend to the rectum, with small vesicular lesions that ulcerate and then resolve over a few days. Subclinical shedding of HSV from rectal lesions is common and has implications for onward transmission of the virus.[11] Clinical symptoms include severe pain, difficulty in passing a bowel movement, tenesmus, discharge, and constitutional symptoms (eg, fever, inguinal lymphadenopathy). Primary infection may be associated with urinary retention, sacral paresthesia or dysesthesia, and short-term impotence.[21]

Conversely, HSV and *T pallidum* infect the stratified squamous epithelium and are commonly seen in the perianal area and at the anal verge. Infections occurring between the anal verge and the anorectal (dentate) line tend to be extremely painful because of the abundance of sensory nerve endings in this area.[11] *T pallidum*, or primary syphilis, may also coexist as a cause of proctitis. Anorectal chancres may go unnoticed by the patient or may be associated with pain or discomfort, itching, bleeding, discharge, and tenesmus.[22] Syphilitic lesions may coexist with HSV and are extremely infectious. The subsequent granulomatous inflammation can lead to rectal masses or widespread maculopapular rash and lesions of the mucous membranes, which may affect the rectum.[23] In the presence of risky sexual practices, there has been an observation of high rates of coinfections as supported by Hascoet and colleagues.[24] In this study, 19% of the 194 MSM enrolled in the study had gonorrhea and chlamydia coinfection, whereas 5.7% had an HIV and syphilis coinfection.[24] The symptoms of many of these infections or coinfections can mimic other conditions that are not STI related. It is therefore imperative that health care professionals caring for MSM patients with anorectal symptoms are aware of the manifestations of different infections that may present in this way. MSM presenting with proctitis need to be tested for the common STIs discussed in this section. Treatment can be started empirically while awaiting the microbiological results, thus reducing inflammation and infection duration, which impedes the patient's ability to further transmit infection.[11]

PATHOPHYSIOLOGY

The anal canal is 2.5 to 3.5 cm in length and IS externally surrounded by internal and external sphincter muscles.[25] The anal canal encompasses columnar and squamous epithelium and is centrally divided by the dentate line. Below the irregularly formed dentate line and extending to the perianus is the squamous epithelium called the andoderm. Andoderm is a highly sensitive area that is similar to normal skin leading to the perianus. The dentate line encapsulates small glands contained in anal valves. Above the dentate line, the anal canal is lined with mucous membranes that contain the area's arterial supply, nerve innervation, lymphatic drainage, and epithelial lining.[25]

Proctitis involves mucosal cell loss within the anal canal and acute inflammation of the lamina propria, a loose connective tissue that lies beneath the epithelium. This inflammatory process also includes the development of eosinophilic crypt abscesses and endothelial edema of the arterioles. In chronic proctitis, dysfunction of the rectal tissue in the anal canal is followed by subsequent fibrosis of connective tissue and endarteritis of the arterioles, which results in mucosal ischemia, friability, bleeding, ulcers, strictures, and fistula formation.

RISK FACTORS

The cause of proctitis stems from either an infectious or a noninfectious pathogen. There are several predisposing factors that increase the likelihood of the onset of proctitis from an infectious pathogen[3,5,25]:

- Ages 15 to 24 years
- MSM
- Multiple anonymous sex partners
- Either receptive or insertive anal sex without a condom
- Presence of another STI
- Positive status for HIV or AIDS

- Substance abuse
- Rectal instrumentation or trauma to the anorectal area

Of these risk factors, the most common mechanism of STI acquisition is anal sex. This widely practiced form of intercourse among heterosexuals and especially MSM is a major risk factor in rectal infections.[25] The understanding of risk factors coupled with epidemiologic data (eg, incidence, prevalence) in a specific geographic setting can equip health care providers with all the knowledge necessary to properly screen those at highest risk for proctitis.

CLINICAL PRESENTATION

The clinical presentation of proctitis caused by an infectious pathogen can often present as vague, nonspecific symptoms. The hallmark symptoms of proctitis typically involve the anorectal area: pain, bleeding, discharge, change in bowel habits, and tenesmus.[3,6,25] Other symptoms, such as abdominal pain or cramping, bloating, flatulence, or mucous in stool, that mimic other gastrointestinal disease processes may be included in a patient's complaint. Clinical presentation and reported symptoms may vary with subsequent visits if not properly treated (**Table 2**). More specifically, LGV-caused proctitis may present asymptomatically or with mucoid or hemorrhagic rectal discharge, anal pain, constipation, fever, or tenesmus. Chronic proctitis presents with rectal bleeding, diarrhea, urgency, tenesmus, incontinence, or pelvic pain. Symptoms may present intermittently and alternate between periods of remissions and relapses. It should be noted that there is a significant overlap in the clinical symptoms of proctitis and common gastrointestinal diseases, particularly irritable bowel syndrome (IBS):

- Abdominal pain or cramping
- Bloating
- Flatulence

Table 2	
Example of variability in patient's history with subsequent visits of untreated proctitis	
Visit 1	Chief complaint: "Lump inside rectum with rectal bleeding." History: 30-y-old man presents with some pain × 1 wk with rectal pain and bleeding. Went to emergency room and treated with pain meds. No fever or chills or sweats. Has been going on and off for more than 2 y. Feels well now. Good health now.
Visit 2 (3 d later)	Chief complaint: "Abdominal pain." History: 30-y-old man presents with complaint of epigastric pain. Describes pain as bloating, cramping, and aching. Pain makes it difficult to sleep. Rates pain as 9/10 and constant. History of kidney stones, IBS, thyroid disease, and foreign travel. Pain increased with defecation. Relieved with hydrocodone use. Denies fever, chills, blood in urine, heartburn, and shortness of breath. Notes: had colonoscopy and esophagogastroduodenoscopy today.
Visit 3 (3 d after visit 2)	Chief complaint: "rectum pain." History: 30-y-old man presents with complaint of abdominal pain with bowel movement. May be injury. Treating with narcotic and laxative.

- Alternating episodes of diarrhea and constipation
- Mucus in the stool

The patient may state that these symptoms improve, worsen, or spontaneously resolve with each clinical presentation. Infectious pathogens will often result in the presence of perianal or rectal ulcers, chancres, condyloma, or tender inguinal lymphadenopathy.[5,6] If not properly diagnosed and treated, symptoms will continue, but the intensity and duration of symptoms may vary with subsequent visits.

LABORATORY TESTS AND FINDINGS

Initial tests should focus on eliminating infectious pathogens as a cause. During the clinical visit, a thorough anal examination should be performed. Commonly, laboratory tests, such as a complete blood count and comprehensive metabolic panel, may be ordered only for results to return negative. Laboratory testing ordered should include tests for STIs, specifically chlamydia and gonorrhea, because those infections can be asymptomatic (**Table 3**).[26] In the case of proctitis, one of these tests will likely be positive. In addition to STIs, MSM with possible proctitis should be tested for HIV and syphilis because of the high risk and likelihood of coinfection. The standard of care for an individual presenting with clinical symptoms of proctitis should include examination by anoscopy.[5] Anorectal exudate observed during the anal examination or anoscopy should be collected for a gram-stained smear to determine the presence of polymorphonuclear leukocytes.[5]

Unfortunately, STI testing is not routinely ordered because of the lack of specificity of the patient's history and normal physical examination findings. Repeated visits may lead health care providers to order other laboratory or diagnostic tests, including but not limited to stool cultures or smears, anoscopy, colonoscopy, biopsy, or serologic markers. These tests will have unremarkable findings leading to diagnoses such as "rectal pain" or "abdominal pain." Additional testing of oral gonorrhea and chlamydia may be warranted for individuals complaining of unresolved sore or "strep" throat. However, proctitis should lead the list of differentials if diagnostic testing reveals the presence of perianal abscesses, fistulae, fissures, or rectal ulcers.

MANAGEMENT AND FOLLOW-UP

Treatment guidelines for proctitis among MSM mirror those for STIs that may present in any individual. However, there are some caveats. The Centers for Disease Control and Prevention (CDC) recommends empirical treatment of proctitis in MSM who have engaged in receptive anal intercourse while awaiting the results of a gram-stained smear or anoscopy.[5] The recommended pharmacologic approach for empirical

Table 3
Laboratory testing for infectious pathogens

Infectious Pathogen	Laboratory Test
N gonorrhoeae	Gram stain, NAAT culture
C trachomatis (LGV)	NAAT, immunofluorescence, culture
C trachomatis (non-LGV)	NAAT, culture
HSV 2	NAAT, viral culture
Syphilis	VDRL, RPR, Treponema pallidum Antibody, immunoglobulin G

Abbreviations: NAAT, Nucleic acid amplification test; RPR, rapid plasma regain; VDRL, Venereal Disease Research Laboratory test.

treatment is Ceftriaxone 250 mg intramuscularly once coupled with Doxycycline 100 mg orally twice a day for a duration of 7 days.[3,5] This treatment ensures that the infectious pathogens gonorrhea and chlamydia are covered. Empirical treatment should also be provided during clinical situations when bloody discharge, perianal ulcers, or mucosal ulcers are found in MSM because this i indicates LGV. This treatment is particularly recommended in the presence of a positive Chlamydia or HIV test. In the presence of clinical symptoms and examination findings that indicate other STIs as possible pathogens, treatment should mirror guidelines for those specific pathogens (**Table 4**).

It is recommended that abstinence from sexual intercourse is strongly encouraged until the completion of at least a 7-day pharmacologic regimen and the resolution of symptoms.[3,5] This recommendation includes the partners of individuals with a confirmed STI or one who is receiving empirical treatment. It is recommended that all partners within a 60-day window be notified, evaluated, tested, and empirically treated for any pathogen in which the individual tested positive. The timeline for follow-up for proctitis in MSM is based on the infectious pathogen being treated and severity of clinical symptoms.[5] In chlamydial or gonococcal proctitis, retesting for the respective pathogen should be performed 3 months after treatment.[3,5]

HUMAN IMMUNODEFICIENCY VIRUS AND PROCTITIS

The presence of an STI increases the likelihood of increased susceptibility or increased infectiousness among MSM. Increased susceptibility means that individuals with an STI are 2 to 5 times more likely to acquire HIV through sexual contact compared with individuals without an STI. Increased infectiousness means that a person living with HIV (PLWH) who has an STI is more likely to transmit HIV through sexual contact compared with a person who does not have HIV. There are 2 mechanisms by which inflammatory processes are triggered that increase susceptibility of HIV acquisition in the presence of STIs: genital and nongenital ulcers. Genital ulcers often present clinically in the presence of syphilis or herpetic infections and result in opportunity for pathogen entry through the genital tract lining or skin. Nonulcerative STIs, such as chlamydia and gonorrhea, increase the concentration of $CD4^+$ cells that can serve as targets for HIV. The presence of an STI in PLWH increases infectiousness because the STI increases the likelihood of HIV being shed in their genital secretions. MSM living with HIV and who have an STI have a median concentration 10 times higher compared

Table 4	
Pharmacologic treatment of proctitis by infectious pathogen	
Infectious Pathogen	**Laboratory Test**
N gonorrhoeae	Ceftriaxone 250 mg intramuscular or cefixime 400 mg orally[a,b]
C trachomatis (LGV)	Doxycycline 100 mg orally twice daily for 3 wk
C trachomatis (non-LGV)	Doxycycline 100 mg orally twice daily for 1 wk
HSV 2	Acyclovir 400 mg orally 3 times daily for 10 d
Syphilis	Penicillin G benzathine 2.4 million units intramuscular once

[a] Consider treatment or LGV as well in addition to this regimen to cover possible coinfection of chlamydia with diagnosis of gonorrhea.
[b] Frequency changes with exposure of unknown duration.

with their counterparts who only have HIV. The higher the median concentration of HIV in genital fluids or semen, the greater the likelihood that HIV will be transmitted to a partner. MSM with a coinfection of HIV and proctitis may present with clinical symptoms, such as bloody discharge, painful perianal ulcers, or mucosal ulcers. Empirical treatment should include a regimen for genital herpes and LGV.[3,25]

COMPLICATIONS OF UNTREATED PROCTITIS

Because of symptoms mirroring those of most gastrointestinal diseases, STI-caused proctitis is often inappropriately treated over a period of time. Asymptomatic presentations, misdiagnosis, and inappropriate treatment have the potential to exacerbate the symptoms of proctitis among MSM, resulting in damage to the rectal and sigmoidal mucosa requiring surgical intervention in cases in which oral medication does not resolve symptoms. Damage caused by the presence of STIs includes the onset of anemia, rectal mucosal ulceration, fistula development, abscesses, and other complications. Untreated proctitis specifically caused by LGV can result in the development of perirectal abscesses, fissures, and stenosis secondary to the obstruction of lymphatic drainage and genital elephantiasis.[18,27,28] Because of the severity of complications, it is vital that all health care professionals are diligent in efforts to prevent and screen for STIs among MSM with rectal complaints.

IMPLICATIONS TO CARE

It is imperative that prevention efforts are implemented for MSM because they are at high risk for proctitis and subsequently HIV. Health care providers must acquire thorough, accurate, and current sexual histories to effectively screen for the presence of STIs in clinical encounters when MSMs present with symptoms indicative of proctitis. Obtaining a sexual history is especially important in MSMs who may be asymptomatic or at high risk for coinfection. The initiative to provide STI prevention, testing, and treatment within the clinical setting is key to providing comprehensive and holistic care to this population. Health care provider's attentiveness to STI epidemiologic trends in their respective geographic area can provide insight into the likelihood of proctitis and HIV in their clinical setting. Specific to HSV, it is critical that individuals are aware of any positive laboratory findings because it is not a curable STI. MSM must take precautionary measures to protect themselves from HIV because of their potentially chronic susceptibility.

The CDC/Health Resources and Services Administration (HRSA) Advisory Committee on HIV/AIDS and STD Prevention recommended the following related to STIs and HIV[29]:

- Early detection and treatment of curable STIs should become a major, explicit component of comprehensive HIV prevention at national, state, and local programs levels.
- Screening and treatment of STIs should be expanded in geographic areas where STIs that increase susceptibility are prevalent, and screening and treatment programs should be expanded.
- Any suspicion or diagnosis of an STI should be tested for HIV.
- Clinical interventions should also target an individual's social, behavioral, or biomedical history.

In addition to these recommendations, it is also critical that providers are attentive to barriers of care that MSM may experience within the clinical setting. Because of the vague, nonspecific symptoms of proctitis coupled with the stigma of being an

MSM, this population often faces barriers related to provider perception and their own comfort level. As the number of subsequent visits increase because of improper treatment, MSM can often be stigmatized as being a "frequent flyer" or "pain seeking." This stigmatization leads to an often-unnecessary stereotype label. In addition, MSM may limit the amount of information disclosed during the clinical visit. This lack of information is related to perceived cultural ideas for health care providers and discomfort with disclosure of personal information related to their unresolved pain. Therefore, the onus is on health care providers to be educated on proctitis symptoms and get a thorough history during the individual's visit with them. Based on the individual's comfort level, health care providers can offer the opportunity for self-collected rectal swabs.[25] Last, counseling addressing safe sex practices is important and should occur with every encounter.

SUMMARY

Proctitis is an often overlooked and misdiagnosed disease that has the potential to negatively impact MSM. Its symptoms are often misleading and result in improper treatment and untimely management. Screening for STIs should be a priority among those presenting with symptoms of proctitis, especially MSM. A thorough sexual history and clinical examination may be a key in the appropriate treatment of a population already facing stigma, stereotypes, and discrimination. It is imperative that all barriers to care, whether by the health care provider or patient, are removed or eliminated to ensure that MSM are receiving comprehensive, holistic care. Preventative strategies within clinical settings should be based on epidemiologic data for the geographic area. Such awareness and prevention strategies are a key to prevention of proctitis and HIV, while positively impacting the health of MSM by limiting the susceptibility and infectiousness of STIs among this group.

DISCLOSURE

The authors have nothing to disclose.

REFERENCES

1. Centers for Disease Control and Prevention. Information for teens: staying healthy and preventing STIs. 2017. Available at: https://www.cdc.gov/std/life-stages-populations/YouthandSTDs-Dec-2017.pdf. Accessed January 14, 2020.
2. Centers for Disease Control and Prevention. Sexually transmitted disease surveillance. 2018. Available at: https://www.cdc.gov/std/stats18/STDSurveillance2018-full-report.pdf. Accessed January 14, 2020.
3. Centers for Disease Control and Prevention. Proctitis, proctocolitis, and enteritis. 2015. Available at: https://www.cdc.gov/std/tg2015/proctitis.htm. Accessed January 14, 2020.
4. Hoentjen F, Rubin DT. Infectious proctitis: when to suspect it is not inflammatory bowel disease. Dig Dis Sci 2012;57(2):269–73.
5. Centers for Disease Control and Prevention. Sexually transmitted diseases treatment guidelines, 2015. MMWR Recomm Rep 2015;64(3):1–137. Available at: https://www.cdc.gov/std/tg2015/tg-2015-print.pdf. Accessed January 14, 2020.
6. Lee KJ, Kim J, Shin DH, et al. Chlamydial proctitis in a young man who has sex with men: misdiagnosed as inflammatory bowel disease. Chonnam Med J 2015; 51(3):139–41.

7. Wu XR, Liu XL, Katz S, et al. Pathogenesis, diagnosis, and management of ulcerative proctitis, chronic radiation proctopathy, and diversion proctitis. Inflamm Bowel Dis 2015;21(3):703–15.
8. Mayo Clinic. Proctitis. 2018. Available at: https://www.mayoclinic.org/diseases-conditions/proctitis/symptoms-causes/syc-20376933. Accessed February 10, 2020.
9. Glotzer DJ, Glick ME, Goldman H. Proctitis and colitis following diversion of the fecal stream. Gastroenterology 1981;80(3):438–41.
10. Carroccio A, Scalici C, Maresi E, et al. Chronic constipation and food intolerance: a model of proctitis causing constipation. Scand J Gastroenterol 2005;40(1): 33–42.
11. Hamlyn E, Taylor C. Sexually transmitted proctitis. Postgrad Med J 2006;82(973): 733–6.
12. Kent C, Chaw J, Wong W, et al. Prevalence of rectal, urethral, and pharyngeal chlamydia and gonorrhea detected in 2 clinical settings among men who have sex with men: San Francisco, California, 2003. Clin Infect Dis 2005;41(1):67–74.
13. El-Dhuwaib Y, Ammori B. Perianal abscess due to Neisseria gonorrhoeae: an unusual case in the post-antibiotic era. Eur J Clin Microbiol Infect Dis 2003;22(7): 422–3.
14. Manavi K, McMillan A, Young H. The prevalence of rectal Chlamydial infection amongst men who have sex with men attending the genitourinary medicine clinic in Edinburgh. Int J STD AIDS 2004;15(3):162–4.
15. Nieuwenhuis R, Ossewaarde J, Gotz H, et al. Resurgence of lymphogranuloma venereum in Western Europe: an outbreak of Chlamydia trachomatis serovar L2 proctitis in the Netherlands among men who have sex with men. Clin Infect Dis 2004;39(7):996–1003.
16. Van der Bij A, Spaargaren J, Morré S, et al. Diagnostic and clinical implications of anorectal lymphogranuloma venereum in men who have sex with men: a retrospective case-control study. Clin Infect Dis 2006;42(2):186–94.
17. Ward H, Martin I, Macdonald N, et al. Lymphogranuloma venereum in the United Kingdom. Clin Infect Dis 2006;44(1):26–32.
18. Lopez-Vicente J, Rodriguez-Alalde D, Hernandez-Villalba L, et al. Proctitis as the clinical presentation of lymphogranuloma venereum, a re-emerging disease in developed countries. Rev Esp Enferm Dig 2014;106(1):59–62.
19. Blank S, Schillinger J, Harbatkin D. Lymphogranuloma venereum in the industrialized world. Lancet 2005;365(9471):1607–8.
20. Solomon L, Cannon MJ, Reyes M. Epidemiology of recurrent genital herpes simplex virus types 1 and 2. Sex Transm Infect 2003;79(6):456–9.
21. Goodell S, Quinn T, Mkrtichian E, et al. Herpes simplex virus proctitis in homosexual men. Clinical, sigmoidoscopic, and histopathological features. N Engl J Med 1983;308(15):868–71.
22. Mindel A, Tovey SJ, Timmins DJ, et al. Primary and secondary syphilis, 20 years' experience. 2. Clinical features. Genitourin Med 1989;65(1):1–3.
23. Bassi O, Cosa G, Colavolpe A, et al. Primary syphilis of the rectum—endoscopic and clinical features. Report of a case. Dis Colon Rectum 1991;34(11):1024–6.
24. Hascoet J, Dahoun M, Cohen M, et al. Clinical diagnostic and therapeutic aspects of 221 consecutive anorectal Chlamydia trachomatis and Neisseria gonorrhoeae sexually transmitted infections among men who have sex with men. Int J Infect Dis 2018;71:9–13.
25. Wilcox C. Evaluation of anorectal symptoms in men who have sex with men. UpToDate. 2019. Available at: https://www-uptodate-com.ckmproxy.vumc.org/contents/

evaluation-of-anorectal-symptoms-in-men-who-have-sex-with-men?search=
proctitis,%20infectious&source=search_result&selectedTitle=2~131&usage_
type=default&display_rank=2#H3401614899. Accessed January 3, 2020.
26. de Vries H, Zingoni A, White J, et al. European Guideline on the management of
proctitis, proctocolitis and enteritis caused by sexually transmissible pathogens.
Int J STD AIDS 2013;25(7):465–74.
27. Pérez-Sánchez L, Hernández-Barroso M, Hernández-Hernández G. Rectal inflammatory stenosis secondary to Chlamydia trachomatis: a case report. Rev
Esp Enferm Dig 2017;109(9):668–9.
28. Workowski KA, Bolan GA, Centers for Disease Control and Prevention. Sexually
transmitted diseases treatment guidelines, 2015. MMWR Recomm Rep 2015;
64(No. RR-03):1–137.
29. Centers for Disease Control and Prevention. HIV prevention through early detection and treatment of other sexually transmitted diseases—United States. Recommendations of the Advisory Committee for HIV and STD prevention. MMWR
Recomm Rep 1998;47(No. RR-12):1–24.

Herpes Simplex Virus
Epidemiology, Diagnosis, and Treatment

Shannon Cole, DNP, APRN-BC

KEYWORDS

- Herpes simplex virus • Sexually transmitted infection • Management

KEY POINTS

- Genital herpes simplex virus (HSV) infections are among the most prevalent sexually transmitted infections in the United States.
- The Centers for Disease Control and Prevention recommendation for clinical diagnosis is confirmation through type-specific virology and type-specific serology tests.
- The diagnosis of herpes can cause life-long psychological complications.

Although most of the key findings related to herpes simplex virus (HSV) infection and treatment have been made in the twentieth century, the first knowledge of HSV can be traced to the ancient Greeks. Hippocrates was the first to describe lesions that could have been attributed to HSV. For centuries, the terminology used by early investigators continued to evolve, because many skin conditions, such as cutaneous lupus, were described as being herpetic. It was not until the nineteenth century that the term herpes was used to describe infections characterized as vesicular appearing for a limited duration.[1]

Genital HSV infections are among the most prevalent sexually transmitted infections (STI) in the United States. Genital HSV continues to be a public health concern because of its recurrent nature and potential for complications. Current treatment is not curative, but rather serves to shorten the duration of symptoms and improve quality of life. Current therapies include episodic treatment and chronic suppressive therapy and are generally well tolerated and effective. This article provides a description of the epidemiology, pathogenesis, clinical features, diagnosis, complications, management, and ethical considerations associated with HSV.

EPIDEMIOLOGY

Genital herpes affects more than 400 million persons worldwide.[2] The Centers for Disease Control and Prevention (CDC) estimates that 776,000 people in the United States

Vanderbilt University School of Nursing, 461 21st Avenue South, 368 Frist Hall, Nashville, TN 37240, USA
E-mail address: shannon.cole@vanderbilt.edu

Nurs Clin N Am 55 (2020) 337–345
https://doi.org/10.1016/j.cnur.2020.05.004
0029-6465/20/© 2020 Elsevier Inc. All rights reserved.
nursing.theclinics.com

acquire new genital herpes infections annually.[3] A 2015 to 2016 National Health and Nutrition Examination Survey among persons aged 14 to 49 years provided national estimates of HSV-1 and HSV-2 antibody prevalence. During 2015 to 2016, the prevalence of HSV-1 and HSV-2 was 47.8% and 11.9%, respectively. This number was lower than the number of cases reported during 1999 to 2000 where the prevalence was 50.4% and 18.0%, respectively. The prevalence of both HSV types increased with age and was higher among women than men. Prevalence of HSV-1 was highest among Mexican Americans and lowest among non-Hispanic white persons. HSV-2 prevalence was highest among non-Hispanic African Americans and lowest among non-Hispanic Asians.[4]

DISEASE PATHOGENESIS

HSV primarily affects the skin and mucus membranes irrespective of the viral type. Biological features unique to HSV include latency and reactivation. Initial exposure to HSV leads to viral invasion of epithelial cells and intracellular replication at the site of primary exposure. After the initial infection, the HSV ascends through the periaxonal sheath of sensory nerves to the sacral ganglia of the hosts nervous system, where the virus replicates and persists in a dormant state and is protected from the host response.[5,6] The sacral ganglia will serve as a reservoir for future outbreaks and subclinical genital shedding.[7] Subsequent outbreaks, caused by a reactivation of latent virus, are usually milder.

There are several stimuli that trigger reactivation of HSV. Neurons in the ganglia may be reactivated by the following:

- Local injury to tissues
- Systemic physical or emotional stress
- Fever
- Microbial infection
- UV exposure
- Hormone imbalances
- Immunosuppression through chemotherapy and body irradiation[8]

HERPES SIMPLEX VIRUS

There are 2 types of HSV: herpes simplex 1 (HSV-1) and herpes simplex 2 (HSV-2). Each type presents differently clinically and varies in severity. HSV-1 commonly causes herpes labialis, herpetic stomatitis, and keratitis. HSV-2 typically causes genital herpes.[9] HSV-2 is transmitted primarily by direct sexual contact with lesions. However, it is estimated that most genital herpes infections are transmitted by persons unaware that they have the infection or who are asymptomatic when transmission occurs.[10] Most genital HSV infections are caused by HSV-2. However, an increasing number are attributable to HSV-1 and are typically less severe and less prone to occurrence (**Table 1**).[11]

Herpes Simplex 1

Infections caused by HSV-1 represent one of the more widespread infections of the orofacial region. Primary HSV-1 infections give rise to mucocutaneous vesicular lesions of the tongue, lips, gingiva, buccal mucosa, and the hard and soft palates. Most HSV-1 infections occur in childhood, with the lifelong potential for symptomatic and asymptomatic viral shedding and in rare cases can lead to more serious complications, such as encephalitis.[12] Recurrent HSV-1 infections of the oral mucosa are

Table 1
Herpes simplex virus types and manifestations

Type	Clinical Manifestations
HSV-1	Gingivostomatitis Keratoconjunctivitis Cutaneous herpes Genital herpes Encephalitis Herpes labialis Meningitis Esophagitis Pneumonia[a] Hepatitis[a]
HSV-2	Genital herpes Cutaneous herpes Gingivostomatitis Neonatal herpes Meningitis Hepatitis[a]

[a] Immunocompromised patients.
Data from Whitley, R.J. and Roizman B. Herpes simplex virus infections. Lancet. 2001 May 12;357(9267):1513-8.

uncommon in otherwise healthy patients. However, immunocompromised patients often experience recurrent, aggressive outbreaks.[13] In addition, although HSV-1 is primarily caused by oral-oral contact, it has the potential to be transmitted through oral sex, causing a genital infection.[12]

Herpes Simplex 2

HSV-2 is an STI and is the leading cause of genital lesions. Primary infection is initiated during sexual contact when the transmitting partner is shedding the virus, often in an asymptomatic fashion.[14] HSV-2 is initiated in genital keratinocytes and may spread to thousands of cells. It increases the risk of human immunodeficiency virus (HIV) acquisition and causes neonatal herpes, a rare infection associated with neurologic impairment and high mortalities, which is transmitted during vaginal delivery through direct mucosal or skin contact.[7]

Risk factors can be categorized as biological or behavioral and can be markers of population subgroups that are likely to have acquired, or are at high risk of acquiring, HSV-2. Major factors associated with HSV-2 include female gender, hormonal contraception, race, history of STIs, increased numbers of sexual partners, and low socioeconomic status or level of education. Age-related risk factors likely reflect the cumulative number of sex partners, age of initiation of sexual activity, and duration of sexual activity. Understanding and identifying these factors may help to direct interventions aimed at reducing HSV-2 transmission and acquisition.[2,15]

TRANSMISSION

HSV infections are transmitted through contact with herpetic lesions, mucosal surfaces, genital secretions, or oral secretions. HSV-1 and HSV-2 can be shed in the absence of lesions. Generally, infection is spread during genital contact with someone who has a genital HSV-2 infection. However, receiving oral sex form a person with HSV-1 can result in acquiring a genital HSV-1 infection. Transmission often occurs from contact with an infected partner without visible lesions or individuals who are un-aware that they are infected. Genital HSV shedding occurs in 10.2% of days in persons with asymptomatic HSV-2 infections, compared with 20.1% of days in those with symptomatic infection.[3]

The average incubation period after exposure is typically 4 days, but may range between 2 and 12 days.[6] Subsequent outbreaks, caused by a reactivation of latent virus, may have a prodrome that is usually milder and heals between 6 and 12 days.[2] Reactivation of latent HSV infection results in symptomatic recurrence of lesions or asymptomatic viral shedding.[16] Reactivation can be triggered by a variety of stimuli and increases lytic gene expression, thus increasing production of the HSV virus, increasing the likelihood of transmission to new hosts.[8] In general, most individuals with symptomatic primary HSV-2 of the genital tract will experience a reoccurrence, with more than one-third experiencing frequent outbreaks in contrast to those infected with HSV-1.[17]

CLINICAL FEATURES

HSV infections are lifelong, highly variable, and characterized by blisters that can rupture and become painful.[4] HSV enters the body during primary infection, and the initial presentation can be severe with painful genital ulcers, dysuria, fever, tender local inguinal lymphadenopathy, and headache.[17] Clustered vesicles may appear on the genitalia, perineum, buttocks, upper thighs, or perianal areas.[2] The infection may also present as mild or subclinical or may be entirely asymptomatic. There are no clear differences in clinical presentation based on the type of infecting virus. However, HSV-1 infections tend to be less severe than HSV-2 infections.[2,18] Patients infected with HSV-2 generally have more outbreaks annually, occurring 4 to 5 times annually compared with a maximum of 1 occurrence for HSV-1.[2]

Symptomatic reoccurrences may be preceded by localized prodromal symptoms that are typically less severe than the primary outbreak and resolve within 5 to 10 days.[13] Prodromal symptoms typically occur up to 48 hours before a subsequent outbreak and may include fever, swollen lymph nodes, headache, myalgia, and itching or tingling of the skin. During this period, lesions develop after viral release from nerve endings in the epithelium.[19]

Symptoms vary between the initial infection and subsequent outbreaks. The virus will remain dormant throughout a person's lifetime with the number of outbreaks decreasing over time. Recurrences are less common in genital HSV-1 than with HSV-2.[19]

The clinical stages of genital HSV are as follows:

Primary genital HSV occurs in patients who have not been exposed to HSV and who have no antibodies to either HSV-1 or HSV-2.

Nonprimary genital HSV occurs with the acquisition of genital HSV-1 in patients who have HSV-2 antibodies, or by the acquisition of genital HSV-2 in patients who have HSV-1 antibodies.

Recurrent genital HSV occurs with reactivation of genital HSV whereby the lesions are the same type as the serum antibodies.

Each designation may be symptomatic or asymptomatic. Asymptomatic infection can only be detected by type-specific serology testing.[20]

DIAGNOSIS

HSV infection is the second most common STI worldwide and the most common cause of genital ulcers in the developed world. As a result of wide variations in manifestations of genital herpes, a pure clinical diagnosis has been shown to have poor sensitivity, making laboratory testing a necessity for confirmation.[21]

Testing to distinguish HSV-1 from HSV-2 is always recommended, because the type of infection affects both prognosis and subsequent counseling.[22] The CDC recommends clinical diagnosis to be confirmed through type-specific virology and type-specific serology tests.[23] HSV-1 and HSV-2 can be detected in lesions of the skin and mucous membranes in patients with lesions secondary to acute infections or in the absence of lesions from genital mucous membranes to verify asymptomatic viral shedding with virology testing.[17] When mucocutaneous lesions are present, the collection of vesicular fluid by swabbing is preferred.[17] Acute genital HSV infections are also diagnosed by laboratory detection of HSV-1 and HSV-2 DNA by means of polymerase chain reaction (PCR). Accurate type-specific HSV serology tests are based on the HSV-specific glycoprotein G2 (HSV-2) and glycoprotein G1 (HSV-1).[23] Type-specific HSV serologic assays are useful for patients with recurrent lesions who have a negative PCR, a clinical diagnosis without laboratory confirmation, or a partner who has genital HSV. HSV serologic testing is also recommended for persons presenting for an STI evaluation, especially those with multiple sex partners.[23]

MANAGEMENT

Evaluation of overall health, along with assessment of clinical signs and symptoms, is essential to the success of HSV management. Management of HSV does not target viral eradication, but rather the attenuation of clinical course, suppression of recurrence, and reduction of viral shedding and complications. In the absence of antiviral therapy, lesions from a primary outbreak will resolve within 3 weeks. Antiviral medications used to manage HSV do not cure infections, but rather modify the clinical course by inhibiting viral replication and subsequent epithelial damage.[5,7] Treatment may be episodic or suppressive.[16]

In general, prevention and treatment of HSV are managed with pharmacologic regimens that work systemically or topically. Systemic medication administration significantly reduces the activation and replication of HSV. Topical medication administration inhibits local replication resulting in reduction of lesions and is typically used to treat oral HSV-1. For topical medication administration, the amount of bioavailable medication is very low secondary to poor percutaneous transport of active ingredients and is a less effective treatment of genital herpes caused by HSV-2.[24]

Three nucleoside analogues approved for HSV treatment are acyclovir, famciclovir, penciclovir, and valacyclovir. Acyclovir may be administered topically or systemically because it can be given via oral and intravenous routes. Penciclovir is a topical treatment used to treat oral herpes and herpes labialis. Famciclovir and valacyclovir are administered systemically. These agents are preferentially taken up by virally infected cells.[25] Nucleoside analogues have proven to be more efficacious and less toxic than idoxuridine and vidarabine, the previous drugs prescribed to treat HSV infections.[26]

Acyclovir, valacyclovir, and famciclovir are effective therapies for genital herpes caused by HSV-1 and HSV-2. They have excellent safety profiles and rarely cause drug-drug interactions or allergic reactions. Drug selection is based on convenience of administration and cost. Intravenous administration of acyclovir is prescribed when the symptoms of genital herpes are severe or are accompanied by complications in patients who are immunocompromised.[16]

Primary genital HSV is associated with more severe and prolonged manifestations than recurrent outbreaks and warrants treatment. Randomized controlled clinical trials have shown that antiviral treatment reduces symptoms and viral shedding with the maximum benefit of treatment when medication is administered within 72 hours after onset of lesions. Valacyclovir has the most convenience dose of 1 g orally twice a day for 7 to 10 days.[16]

Patients with symptomatic recurrences of genital herpes can receive episodic or suppressive therapy. Episodic therapy is typically prescribed for 1 to 5 days, and suppressive therapy is given daily to reduce the frequency of symptomatic recurrences. Acyclovir, valacyclovir, and famciclovir have similar efficacy for recurrences. However, famciclovir has the most convenient regimen with a dose of 1 g orally every 12 hours for 2 days.[16]

Management of HSV also includes prevention. Preventive strategies aimed at reduction of transmission include education regarding the contagious nature of the disease, efficacy of barrier techniques such as condoms in preventing viral transmission, asymptomatic viral shedding, and avoidance of triggers. In patients who have symptomatic viral shedding, the most effective strategy is abstinence from sexual activity. Postinfection deterrence strategies include episodic and suppressive therapies aimed at reducing the severity, duration, and recurrence of symptoms, along with preventing transmission to uninfected partners.[2,5]

COMPLICATIONS

Persons infected with HSV-2 have a 3-fold risk of acquiring HIV,[2,3] related to broken skin, or lymphocytes at the eruption site facilitating HIV invasion during sexual contact.[2] In addition, genital herpes triggers an inflammatory process that increases the number of target cells for HIV entry (CD4 cells) in the genital mucosa.[3] Local activation of HIV replication at the site of genital herpes in persons with both HIV and HSV-2 will increase the risk that HIV will be transmitted during contact with the mouth, vagina, or rectum of an HIV-uninfected sex partner.[27]

Worldwide, more than half of individuals infected with HIV will also have HSV-2 with the risk of HIV acquisition being 3 times higher in women infected with HSV-2. Genital lesions facilitate HIV acquisition because of disruptions of the skin and mucosa; however, HSV suppression treatment has not been shown to prevent HIV transmission. HSV-2 infection may accelerate HIV disease and increase viral load, and acyclovir has been shown to slow HIV progression in individuals coinfected with HIV and HSV-2.[28]

Recurrent HSV infection is a major cause of morbidity and mortality for immunocompromised patients who experience frequent, persistent, severe recurrences of HSV-1 and HSV-2. Local mucocutaneous oral or genital disease may become chronic and more severe than typical disease in immunocompetent persons, depending on the level of immune function. Typically, there is a longer duration of viral shedding, and lesions are not strictly limited to oral or genital areas and may occur on digits or the face. Numerous immunologic and clinical factors, in combination, provide an opportunity for HSV to become resistant to antiviral therapy, such as a deficit in HSV-specific cell-mediated immunity.[5,29]

Neonatal herpes is a devastating and often fatal consequence of HSV transmission to neonates. Neonates may acquire HSV infections in utero, or during the intrapartum or postpartum stages, with transmission through contact with vaginal secretions containing HSV during the intrapartum period as the most common mode.[5,9] The risk of transmission is significantly higher in mothers experiencing a primary outbreak. Although cesarean delivery has proven to be effective in preventing transmission, neonatal HSV cases have been reported in mothers who had premature rupture of membranes before cesarean delivery.[30] Neonatal HSV causes significant morbidity and mortality. However, with appropriate diagnosis and suppressive therapy, outcomes can be drastically improved.

HSV is typically a self-limited infection and not usually considered life threatening. In rare instances, fatal complications may arise. Neonates and immunocompromised individuals are at a greater risk for developing poor outcomes.

ETHICAL CONSIDERATIONS

Patients are often distressed when the initial diagnosis is made secondary to the fact the HSV is not curable. Reassurance should be given that HSV is manageable and will not majorly impact sexuality. Despite reassurance, feelings of anger, shame, depression, and fear of rejection from sexual partners are common. Because of the sensitive nature and need for specific patient teaching, justice should be paired with autonomy. Justice refers to the element of fairness with regard to medical decisions and treatments, whereas autonomy refers to allowing decision making to be free from coercion. Clinicians should spend the necessary time to educate patients and their partners as to how to prevent transmission and manage disease (justice), and be free to decide how they want to proceed with both episodic and suppressive treatments (autonomy).

Aspects of genital herpes may affect adolescents and young adults differently when compared with older adults. A major concern for adolescents is seeking care without parental knowledge, which may result in a delay of treatment. For both groups, care may be delayed because of confidentiality concerns, discomfort in discussing sexual experiences, and anxiety.[31] Clinicians should be aware of these barriers and be sensitive to them during the patient interview.

SUMMARY

HSV is a common sexually transmitted disease worldwide. Although HSV-2 is typically the causative agent in most cases, HSV-1 is associated with an increasing number of cases. HSV infections are categorized as primary or recurrent, and clinical manifestations are highly variable. The initial presentation is usually severe with painful ulcers and constitutional symptoms. However, some patients may be asymptomatic or experience mild symptoms. Clinical recurrences are common and typically less severe and can be triggered by assaults to the primary immune system. Diagnosis is confirmed by PCR and type-specific serologic tests, and treatment can be episodic or suppressive. HSV treatment is not curative, but the vast systemic and topical medications available aid in management of the virus and prevention of symptomatic outbreaks. Patient teaching on prevention of HSV is the key for health care providers to use in order to reduce the prevalence of HSV and decrease the physical and psychosocial complications that accompany the HSV virus.

DISCLOSURE

The author has nothing to disclose.

REFERENCES

1. Roizman B, Whitley RJ. The nine ages of herpes simplex virus. Herpes 2001; 8(1):23–6.
2. Groves MJ. Genital herpes: a review. Am Fam Physician 2016;93(11):928–34.
3. Prevention, C.f.D.C.a.. Genital herpes–CDC fact sheet (detailed). Available at: https://www.cdc.gov/std/herpes/stdfact-herpes-delatiled.ttm.

4. McQuillan G, Kruszon-Moran D, Flagg EW, et al. Prevalence of herpes simplex virus type 1 and type 2 in persons aged 14-49: United States, 2015-2016. NCHS Data Brief 2018;(304):1–8.
5. Fatahzadeh M, Schwartz RA. Human herpes simplex virus infections: epidemiology, pathogenesis, symptomatology, diagnosis, and management. J Am Acad Dermatol 2007;57(5):737–63 [quiz: 764–6].
6. Kimberlin DW, Rouse DJ. Clinical practice. Genital herpes. N Engl J Med 2004; 350(19):1970–7.
7. Johnston C, Corey L. Current concepts for genital herpes simplex virus infection: diagnostics and pathogenesis of genital tract shedding. Clin Microbiol Rev 2016; 29(1):149–61.
8. Stoeger T, Adler H. "Novel" triggers of herpesvirus reactivation and their potential health relevance. Front Microbiol 2018;9:3207.
9. Lane K, editor. The Merk manual of diagnosis and therapy. 20 edition. Kenilworth (NJ): Merk Sharp & Dohme Corp; 2018.
10. Workowski KA, Bolan GA, Centers for Disease Control and Prevention. Sexually transmitted diseases treatment guidelines, 2015. MMWR Recomm Rep 2015; 64(RR-03):1–137.
11. Whitley RJ, Roizman B. Herpes simplex virus infections. Lancet 2001;357(9267): 1513–8.
12. Looker KJ, Magaret AS, May MT, et al. Global and regional estimates of prevalent and incident herpes simplex virus type 1 infections in 2012. PLoS One 2015; 10(10):e0140765.
13. Arduino PG, Porter SR. Herpes simplex virus type 1 infection: overview on relevant clinico-pathological features. J Oral Pathol Med 2008;37(2):107–21.
14. Schiffer JT, Swan DA, Prlic M, et al. Herpes simplex virus-2 dynamics as a probe to measure the extremely rapid and spatially localized tissue-resident T-cell response. Immunol Rev 2018;285(1):113–33.
15. Wald A. Herpes simplex virus type 2 transmission: risk factors and virus shedding. Herpes 2004;11(Suppl 3):130A–7A.
16. Gnann JW Jr, Whitley RJ. CLINICAL PRACTICE. Genital herpes. N Engl J Med 2016;375(7):666–74.
17. Sauerbrei A. Optimal management of genital herpes: current perspectives. Infect Drug Resist 2016;9:129–41.
18. Bernstein DI, Bellamy AR, Hook EW 3rd, et al. Epidemiology, clinical presentation, and antibody response to primary infection with herpes simplex virus type 1 and type 2 in young women. Clin Infect Dis 2013;56(3):344–51.
19. Mospan CM, Cluck D. Prevention and management of genital herpes. US Pharmacist 2016;41(4):30–3.
20. Albrecht MA. Epidemiology, clinical manifestations, and diagnosis of genital herpes simplex virus infection. UpToDate; 2019.
21. Patwardhan V, Bhalla P. Role of type-specific herpes simplex virus-1 and 2 serology as a diagnostic modality in patients with clinically suspected genital herpes: a comparative study in Indian population from a tertiary care hospital. Indian J Pathol Microbiol 2016;59(3):318–21.
22. LeGoff J, Pere H, Belec L. Diagnosis of genital herpes simplex virus infection in the clinical laboratory. Virol J 2014;11:83.
23. Prevention, C.f.D.C.a.. 2015 sexually transmitted diseases treatment guidelines. Available at: https://www.cdc.gov/std/tg2015/herpes.htm. Accessed December 27, 2019.
24. Angle E.N. Treatment of virus-based diseases of the skin. 2019, Google Patents.

25. Poole CL, Kimberlin DW. Antiviral approaches for the treatment of herpes simplex virus infections in newborn infants. Annu Rev Virol 2018;5(1):407–25.
26. James SH, Prichard MN. Current and future therapies for herpes simplex virus infections: mechanism of action and drug resistance. Curr Opin Virol 2014;8:54–61.
27. Barnabas RV, Celum C. Infectious co-factors in HIV-1 transmission herpes simplex virus type-2 and HIV-1: new insights and interventions. Curr HIV Res 2012;10(3):228–37.
28. Emre S, Akkus A. Genital herpes. 2017. p. 49.
29. Levin MJ, Bacon TH, Leary JJ. Resistance of herpes simplex virus infections to nucleoside analogues in HIV-infected patients. Clin Infect Dis 2004; 39(Supplement_5):S248–57.
30. Pinninti SG, Kimberlin DW. Neonatal herpes simplex virus infections. Semin Perinatol 2018;42(3):168–75.
31. Roberts C. Genital herpes in young adults: changing sexual behaviours, epidemiology and management. Herpes 2005;12(1):10–4.

Pharmacology Update for the Treatment of Hepatitis C Virus

Leslie Hopkins, DNP, FNP-C, ANP-C*, Travis Dunlap, PhD, ANP-C,
Holly Cline, MSN, ANP-C

KEYWORDS

- Hepatitis C virus • Adults • Direct-acting antivirals • Cirrhosis
- Chronic kidney disease

KEY POINTS

- Hepatitis C is the most common blood-borne infection in the United States.
- New cases of hepatitis C have been increasing since 2010.
- Hepatitis C can now be cured with direct-acting antiviral medications.
- It is of utmost importance that clinicians are up to date on the latest treatment options for patients infected with hepatitis C.

INTRODUCTION

The hepatitis C virus (HCV) is the most common blood-borne infection in the United States.[1] HCV is a viral infection of the liver that can be acute and chronic. The World Health Organization (WHO) estimates there are 71 million cases of HCV worldwide.[2] According to the Centers for Disease Control and Prevention (CDC), new cases of acute HCV in the United States have been steadily increasing since 2010.[3] An estimated 2 million to 3 million individuals in the United States have chronic HCV, half of whom are unaware of the infection.[4] Acute HCV can be asymptomatic, often becoming chronic. It takes only a small amount of blood to transmit the virus, and it is contracted most often via injected drug use. Although there is no vaccine for the prevention of infection, chronic HCV can be treated and cured. Untreated HCV can lead to cirrhosis and is the leading cause of liver cancer.[2] Because infection rates are increasing, it is important that health care providers know the risk factors, pathophysiology of the disease, proper diagnostic testing, and appropriate medical treatment.

Vanderbilt University School of Nursing, 461 21st Avenue South, Nashville, TN 37240, USA
* Corresponding author.
E-mail address: leslie.hopkins@Vanderbilt.edu

Nurs Clin N Am 55 (2020) 347–359
https://doi.org/10.1016/j.cnur.2020.06.008
0029-6465/20/© 2020 Elsevier Inc. All rights reserved.

nursing.theclinics.com

PATHOPHYSIOLOGY

Researchers in the 1970s observed that a significant amount of hepatitis cases resulting from blood transfusions were not hepatitis A or hepatitis B viruses.[5] The distinct HCV was eventually discovered in 1989.[6] This discovery has enabled the development of effective methods of diagnosing, treating, and managing HCV infections. To better understand HCV infections, it is necessary to understand the pathophysiology of the disease.

Virology of the Hepatitis C Virus

The HCV belongs to the Flaviviridae family and is the only member of the genus Hepacivirus.[7] The virus is a spherical, positive-sense, RNA virus that measures 40 nm to 80 nm in diameter.[8] Positive-sense describes how DNA or RNA strands translate genetic sequences into a protein. The single RNA strand contains approximately 9600 nucleotide bases.[9]

There are 7 known genotypes (1–7) with most research focusing on genotypes 1 to 6 because genotype 7 has only been isolated once in a few African individuals living in Canada.[10] Within the 6 main genotypes, more than 70 subtypes have been found, with genotype 1 being the most prevalent, causing between 40% and 50% of HCV infections worldwide, including the United States.[7,9] This vast amount of genetic variation arises from HCV's innately high rate of mutation, which is further expanded by the presence of quasispecies.[8]

Quasispecies are closely related, but heterogeneous, sequences of HCV RNA within a single infected person that arise from mutations that occur during viral replication.[7] Individuals with chronic HCV infections produce 10^{12} quasispecies daily because of this extremely high rate of replication and translational errors that provides immense genetic diversity.[9] As a result of this diversity, the HCV is able to rapidly adapt to the body's innate and adaptive immune system response as well antiviral drugs.[8]

Hepatitis C Virus Transmission

There are 2 main modes of HCV transmission, percutaneous (blood borne) and nonpercutaneous routes. Percutaneous routes of HCV transmission include blood transfusions, injection drug use, accidental needle sticks in a health care setting, and chronic hemodialysis. Nonpercutaneous routes of HCV transmission include vertical transmission from mother to infant and high-risk sexual practices.

Percutaneous transmission

The patient population bearing the greatest prevalence of HCV infections worldwide is persons who inject drugs (PWID). It is estimated that 67% of PWID are living with HCV infection and this is responsible for almost 70% of all new HCV infections.[11] It is estimated that most PWID who share needles will test positive for HCV within 6 months of starting.[7] Before the advent of improved diagnostic testing, blood transfusions were another prominent cause of HCV infection. Now, only 1 case occurs in every 2 million units transfused.[7] Chronic hemodialysis is now the second most common route for percutaneous transmission, and it is estimated that less than 10% of individuals on dialysis test positive for HCV.[7] However, this frequency increases to between 55% and 85% in Jordan, Saudi Arabia, Iran.[7]

Nonpercutaneous transmission

In a meta-analysis by Benova and colleagues,[12] the vertical risk of HCV transmission was determined to be 5.8% for pregnant women who were human immunodeficiency virus (HIV) negative and 10.8% for HIV-positive pregnant women. The high-risk sexual practice that has the highest incidence is anal sex in men who have sex with men (MSM) that causes trauma to the anal mucosa.[11] It is estimated that between 5% and 10% of HIV-positive MSM test positive for HCV.[13] This finding contrasts with HIV-negative MSM, where the prevalence was noted to be 1.5%.[13]

Hepatitis C Virus Lifecycle

HCVs are known as hepatotropic because they have a greater affinity for hepatocytes in the liver than other cells in the body. Although hepatocytes are the most frequent site for HCV replication, immune cells such as B cells, T cells, monocytes, and dendritic cells are also hosts for HCV replication.[7] After initial binding to the host cell (**Fig. 1**), the HCV particle is thought to form receptor complexes by interacting with 4 host cell membrane proteins.[14] These proteins are scavenger receptor class B type 1 (SRB1), cluster of differentiation 81 (CD81), claudin 1 (CLDN1), and occludin (OCLN).[14] In step 1, the formation of the receptor complexes allows the HCV particle to enter the host cell by receptor-mediated endocytosis.[14] In step 2, the viral RNA genome is released into the cytoplasm and translated at the rough endoplasmic reticulum (ER) into mature viral proteins.[14] In step 2, these proteins, in conjunction with host cell factors, stimulate the formation of the membranous web that is composed of vesicles as well as lipid droplets.[14] In step 4, RNA replication occurs at an unknown site within the membranous web and produces a negative-sense copy [(−)RNA], which serves as a template to produce vast amounts of positive-sense RNA [(+)RNA].[14] In step 5, production of HCV particles likely originates near the ER and lipid droplets where core protein and viral RNA accumulate.[14] Lipoprotein synthesis in

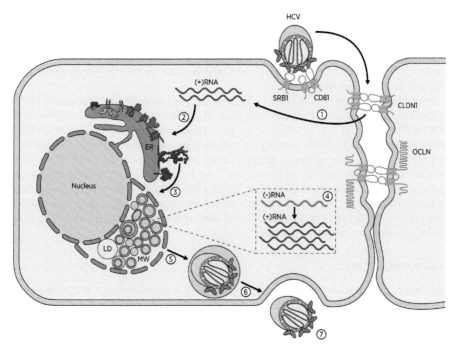

Fig. 1. Initial binding to the host cell. CD81, cluster of differentiation 81; CLDN1, claudin 1; ER, endoplasmic reticulum; LD, lipid droplet; MW, membranous web; OCLN, occluding; SRB1, scavenger receptor class B type 1.

the ER is responsible for producing lipids that form the HCV envelope.[14] In step 6, these lipid-packaged HCV particles are thought to be released via the secretory pathway.[14] In step 7, the ensuing HCV lipoviral particle is then able to travel through the bloodstream and infect other host cells by binding with a low-density lipoprotein receptor found on SRB1.[14]

Chronic Effects of Hepatitis C Virus Infection

In response to HCV infection, the affected hepatocytes activate the innate immune system by inducing the release of interferons (IFNs), specifically, IFN-β.[15] One function of IFN-β is to inhibit viral replication within the affected cells.[15] Another function of IFN-β is to promote the production of chemokines and cytokines that activate the adaptive immune system, which creates a proinflammatory state as long as the HCV infection is present.[15]

An HCV infection lasting more than 6 months is considered to be a chronic infection and intrinsic clearance of HCV is unusual after this time.[15] Because of chronic hepatic inflammation, cellular changes occur, including fibrogenesis, where hepatic stellate cells differentiate to become myofibroblasts.[16] In turn, the myofibroblasts produce excessive amounts of extracellular matrices consisting mainly of collagen.[17] This chronic proinflammatory state directly results in creating the environment that leads to 3 significant forms of liver injury and disease:

- Fibrosis
- Cirrhosis
- Hepatocellular carcinoma (HCC)

Liver fibrosis is a consequence of chronic hepatic inflammation and the subsequent attempt by the immune system to repair the affected areas, which eventually leads to liver cirrhosis over approximately 20 years.[2,17] Cirrhosis is characterized by advanced, diffuse fibrosis with the presence of benign hepatocellular nodules without fibrosis, often referred to as regenerative nodules.[18] Clinical presentation of cirrhosis includes portal hypertension that can cause complications such as ascites, esophageal varices, and encephalopathy.[18]

A third disease that results from fibrosis related to chronic HCV infection is HCC, which may develop in a cirrhotic liver over 20 to 40 years.[5] The development of HCC is multifactorial and is affected by both direct and indirect effects of chronic HCV infection. Direct effects include the inhibition of host cell apoptosis and generation of reactive oxygen species, which is associated with increased risk of somatic mutations and chromosomal abnormalities.[19] An indirect effect stimulating the development of HCC includes the chronic production of proinflammatory chemicals, including INF-γ, that create a tumor-promoting environment.[19] An additional indirect effect is the prolonged but impaired T-cell and antibody response stemming from the HCV's ability to avoid apoptosis.[19]

DIAGNOSTIC TESTING

It is important that health care providers know who is at risk for HCV and screen patients appropriately. Those at risk include individuals born between 1945 and 1965; current or past injection drug users; recipients of blood products; health care workers; chronic hemodialysis patients; HIV-positive individuals; children born to HCV-positive mothers; incarcerated individuals; intranasal drug users; and those getting tattoos in unregulated locations.[1,3] Screening for HCV protects the public health and decreases morbidity and mortality.

Screening for HCV for the detection of anti-HCV antibodies is the first step. A negative anti-HCV antibody test means no further testing needs to be done. Positive HCV antibody testing indicates current (acute or chronic) HCV infection. As such, a positive antibody test requires a confirmation quantitative serum HCV RNA test by polymerase chain reaction for viral load.[20] HCV can be tested via an oral swab. This testing method is convenient and cost-efficient, and is helpful with high-risk populations in whom serum testing may not be the most effective first step. Positive HCV oral swab testing must be followed with a serum antibody test and an HCV RNA test (**Fig. 2**).[20]

Individuals with positive HCV antibodies whose HCV RNA test is negative may not have generated a significant viral load yet and should be tested again in 3 to 6 months.[1,3,4] Persons with active HCV have both positive anti-HCV antibodies and positive HCV RNA tests[1,3,4] (**Table 1**).

Before treatment of active HCV begins, individuals should have additional testing completed. Baseline routine blood testing should include a complete metabolic panel with particular attention to alanine aminotransferase (ALT), aspartate aminotransferase (AST), albumin, bilirubin, alkaline phosphatase (ALP), international normalized ratio (INR), complete blood count with differential, and an estimated glomerular filtration rate and genotyping.[4] In addition, because of the risk of coinfection, individuals should be tested for HIV, hepatitis A virus (HAV), and hepatitis B virus (HBV). If testing is negative, HAV and HBV vaccinations should be administered.[4]

UPDATED GUIDELINES FOR PHARMACOLOGIC TESTING
Goals of Therapy

Over the past decade, the treatment of chronic HCV has undergone a drastic evolution. The highly effective HCV protease inhibitors are the newest direct-acting

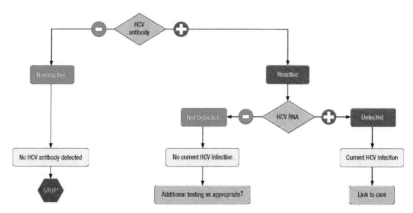

Fig. 2. Recommended testing sequence for identifying current HCV infection. [a] For persons who might have been exposed to HCV within the past 6 months, testing for HCV RNA or follow-up testing for HCV antibody is recommended. For persons who are immunocompromised, testing for HCV RNA can be considered. [b] To differentiate past, resolved HCV infection from biologic false positivity for HCV antibody, testing with another HCV antibody assay can be considered. Repeat HCV RNA testing if the person tested is suspected to have had HCV exposure within the past 6 months or has clinical evidence of HCV disease, or if there is concern regarding the handling or storage of the test specimen. (*From* CDC. Testing for HCV Infection: An update of guidance for clinicians and laboratorians. MMWR 2013;62(18). Available at: https://www.cdc.gov/hepatitis/hcv/pdfs/hcv_flow.pdf. With permission.)

Table 1
Interpretation of results of tests for hepatitis C virus infection and further actions

Test Outcome	Interpretation	Further Actions
HCV antibody nonreactive	No HCV antibody detected	Sample can be reported as nonreactive for HCV antibody. No further action required If recent exposure in person tested is suspected, test for HCV RNA[a]
HCV antibody reactive	Presumptive HCV infection	A repeatedly reactive result is consistent with current HCV infection, or past HCV infection that has resolved, or biological false-positivity for HCV antibody. Test for HCV RNA to identify current infection
HCV antibody reactive, HCV RNA detected	Current HCV infection	Provide person tested with appropriate counseling and link person tested to care and treatment[b]
HCV antibody reactive, HCV RNA not detected	No current HCV infection	No further action required in most cases If distinction between true positivity and biological false-positivity for HCV antibody is desired, and if sample is repeatedly reactive in the initial test, test with another HCV antibody assay In certain situations,[c] follow up with HCV RNA testing and appropriate counseling

[a] If HCV RNA testing is not feasible and person tested is not immunocompromised, do follow-up testing for HCV antibody to show seroconversion. If the person tested is immunocompromised, consider testing for HCV RNA.

[b] It is recommended before initiating antiviral therapy to retest for HCV RNA in a subsequent blood sample to confirm HCV RNA positivity.

[c] If the person tested is suspected of having HCV exposure within the past 6 months, or has clinical evidence of HCV disease, or if there is concern regarding the handling or storage of the test specimen.

From CDC. Testing for HCV infection: An update of guidance for clinicians and laboratorians. MMWR 2013;62(18). Available at: https://www.cdc.gov/hepatitis/hcv/pdfs/hcv_graph.pdf. With permission.

antivirals (DAAs) that have the capacity to achieve sustained virologic response (SVR) with only 8 to 12 weeks of treatment.[3] Sustained virologic response is defined as the absence of a detectable virus after 12 weeks of therapy.[21] Regardless of genotype, 90% of chronic HCV infections can be cured with this shorter and more effective treatment regimen.[3] The National Academies of Science, Engineering, and Medicine have a national goal to decrease the number of chronic HCV infections by 90% before the year 2030.[22] With this goal in mind, the American Association for the Study of Liver Diseases (AASLD) and the Infectious Diseases Society of America (IDSA) have developed guidelines to simplify chronic HCV treatment of treatment-naive and treatment-experienced patients in hopes that it will expand the number of health care professionals willing to prescribe these new DAAs.[23] Because the goal of the AASLD/IDSA guidelines is to increase the numbers of providers treating chronic HCV, the treatment regimens discussed here focus on individuals with HCV infections who do not have comorbid HBV or HIV infections.[24,25]

Treatment Indications

At present, there are only guidelines for treatment of individuals with chronic HCV infections. New treatment guidelines recommend no treatment of acute HCV infections because 20% to 25% of individuals with acute infections clear the virus naturally and have no detectable viral load.[2] Patients with acute HCV infections should have a follow-up HCV RNA 6 months after first determining HCV-positive status because an HCV infection is considered chronic if an HCV RNA has a positive viral load for more than 6 months.[26] Once a patient is determined to have a detectable viral load for more than 6 months, the patient is considered eligible for the treatment of chronic HCV.[24]

Pharmacologic Regimens

Guidelines for treatment-naive patients without cirrhosis
For patients that are treatment naive without cirrhosis, the AASLD/IDSA recommend following a simplified HCV treatment regimen. The recommendations for the simplified regimen are treatment with glecaprevir (300 mg)/pibrentasvir (120 mg) with food for a duration of 8 weeks or sofosbuvir (400 mg)/velpatasvir (100 mg) for a duration of 12 weeks.[24] Twelve weeks after completion of therapy, a quantitative RNA analysis and hepatic function panel should be assessed to determine whether HCV RNA is undetectable, which is known as virologic cure SVR.[24]

A liver biopsy is not necessary for determining whether cirrhosis is present.[26] Guidelines recommend that, if any screening test shows evidence of cirrhosis, the simplified regimen should be avoided.[24] Some common results that would be considered evidence of cirrhosis include Fibrosis-4 score greater than 3.25, AST to platelet ratio index greater than 2.0, platelet count less than 150,000/mm, or a Fibroscan stiffness greater than 12.5 kPa.[24] Individuals not eligible for a simplified treatment regimen include those with a prior history of HCV treatment, history of cirrhosis, prior history of liver transplant, HIV-positive or hepatitis B surface antigen (HBsAg)–positive status, end-stage renal disease, and individuals who are pregnant.[26]

Guidelines for treatment-experienced patients without cirrhosis
For patients who do not meet the criteria for a simplified treatment regimen, because prior treatment did not achieve cure SVR, the recommended guidelines vary based on genotype and cirrhosis status (**Table 2**).[25]

Table 2
Summary of guidelines for experience patients without cirrhosis by genotype

Genotype	Medication Options	Number of Weeks of Treatment
1a and b	Elbasvir/grazoprevir	12
	Glecaprevir/pibrentasvir	8
	Ledipasvir/sofosbuvir	12
	Sofosbuvir/velpatasvir	12
1a and b, subtype NS3	Glecaprevir/pibrentasvir	12
	Ledipasvir/sofosbuvir	12
	Sofosbuvir/velpatasvir	12
1a and b, subtype non-NS5A	Sofosbuvir (400 mg)/velpatasvir (100 mg)/ voxilaprevir (100 mg)	12
1a and b, subtype NS5A	Sofosbuvir (400 mg)/velpatasvir (100 mg)/ voxilaprevir (100 mg)	12
2	Glecaprevir/pibrentasvir	8
	Sofosbuvir/velpatasvir	12
3	Daily fixed-dose combination of sofosbuvir (400 mg)/velpatasvir (100 mg) without baseline Y93H RAS to velpatasvir	12
4	Elbasvir/grazoprevir	12
	Glecaprevir/pibrentasvir	8
	Ledipasvir/sofosbuvir	12
	Sofosbuvir/velpatasvir	12
5 and 6	Glecaprevir/pibrentasvir	8

Retreatment of persons in whom prior therapy failed. Hepatitis C guidance: AASLD-IDSA recommendations for testing, managing, and treating adults infected with hepatitis C virus.

Abbreviation: RAS, resistance-associated substitution.

Adapted from American Association for the Study of Liver Diseases/ Infectious Diseases Society of America HCV Guidance Panel. Retreatment of persons in whom prior therapy failed. Hepatitis C guidance: AASLD-IDSA recommendations for testing, managing, and treating adults infected with hepatitis C virus. Available at: https://www.hcvguidelines.org/Treatment-Experienced. Published 2019. Accessed November 25, 2019. With permission.

Treatment recommendations for patients with decompensated cirrhosis

Patients with HCV infection who also have moderate or severe decompensated cirrhosis should be referred to a hepatologist within a transplant center.[27] Most patients receiving DAA therapy see marked improvement in clinical indicators of liver disease after 12 weeks of treatment.[27] However, these improvements may not be enough and may necessitate liver transplant to avoid further liver-related complications, including death.[27] At this time, there are no predictors of improvement or decline, although outcomes are correlated with severity of underlying liver disease. For this reason, some patients benefit more from liver transplant than DAA therapy (**Table 3**).[27]

Guidelines for Treatment of Unique Populations

Treatment recommendations for hepatitis C virus/human immunodeficiency virus coinfection

HCV/HIV coinfected individuals are at a greater risk for HCV-related complications. Overall, the mortality is much higher for HCV/HIV coinfected individuals.[3] Advanced liver fibrosis and liver cirrhosis are much more likely in coinfected patients, as is

Table 3
Summary of guidelines for experienced patients with cirrhosis by genotype

Genotype	Medication Options	Number of Weeks of Treatment
1a and b	Elbasvir/grazoprevir	12
	Glecaprevir/pibrentasvir	12
	Sofosbuvir/velpatasvir	12
2	Glecaprevir/pibrentasvir	16
	Sofosbuvir/velpatasvir	12
3	Glecaprevir/pibrentasvir	16
	Sofosbuvir/velpatasvir	12
4	Elbasvir/grazoprevir	12
	Glecaprevir/pibrentasvir	12
	Sofosbuvir/velpatasvir	12
5 and 6	Glecaprevir/pibrentasvir	12
	Ledipasvir/sofosbuvir	12
	Sofosbuvir/velpatasvir	12

Patients with decompensated cirrhosis. Hepatitis C guidance: AASLD-IDSA recommendations for testing, managing, and treating adults infected with HCV.

Adapted from American Association for the Study of Liver Diseases/ Infectious Diseases Society of America HCV Guidance Panel. Patients with decompensated cirrhosis. Hepatitis C guidance: AASLD-IDSA recommendations for testing, managing, and treating adults infected with hepatitis C virus Web site. https://www.hcvguidelines.org/unique-populations/decompensated-cirrhosis. Published 2019. Accessed January 7, 2019. With permission.

multiorgan failure.[3] For these reasons, it is important that HCV/HIV coinfected patients receive prompt and appropriate treatment to prevent complications.[28] One of the most complex issues when treating HCV/HIV coinfection is navigating the possible complex drug-drug interactions between DAAs and antiretroviral medications. Once the drug interactions have been recognized and managed, the AASLD-IDSA guidelines recommend those individuals who are HCV/HIV coinfected should be managed using the same guidelines in those without HIV infection.[28] The guidelines do provide regimens that are not recommended for patients with HCV/HIV coinfection (**Table 4**).[28]

Because modes of transmission are similar, HBV is common in patients with HCV/ HIV coinfection. Thus, screening for HBV immunity is imperative.[28] For HCV/HIV coinfected individuals with confirmed history of HBV, there have been case reports of HBV reactivation in patients who are on DAAs without active HBV agents.[29] For this reason, all patients initiating HCV DAA therapy should be assessed for HBV coinfection with HBsAg, hepatitis B surface antibody, and hepatitis B core antibodies testing.[29] Confirmation of HBV infection in an HCV/HIV coinfected individual requires additional treatment with an antiretroviral HBV agent.[29]

Treatment recommendation for renal impairment

HCV infection is linked to 43% increased risk of the development of chronic kidney disease (CKD).[30] There is a high risk of progression to end-stage renal disease in individuals with both chronic HCV and CKD, making early detection and treatment vital.[3] At present, there are no recommendations for dose adjustment of DAAs when using recommended treatment regimens for individuals with stage 1, 2, and 3 CKD.[30] Recommendations for stage 4 and 5 are listed in **Table 5**.[30]

Monitoring During Treatment

Monitoring is an essential part of managing chronic HCV to safely achieve cure SVR.[31] Regular clinic visits during treatment are recommended to ensure patient adherence,

Table 4
Regimens not recommended for patients with human immunodeficiency virus/hepatitis C virus coinfection

Not Recommended	Rating
Antiretroviral treatment interruption to allow HCV therapy is not recommended	III, A
Elbasvir/grazoprevir should not be used with cobicistat, efavirenz, etravirine, nevirapine, or any HIV protease inhibitor	III, B
Glecaprevir/pibrentasvir should not be used with atazanavir, efavirenz, etravirine, nevirapine, or ritonavir-containing antiretroviral regimens	III, B
Sofosbuvir/velpatasvir should not be used with efavirenz, etravirine, or nevirapine	III, B
Sofosbuvir/velpatasvir/voxilaprevir should not be used with efavirenz, etravirine, nevirapine, ritonavir-boosted atazanavir, or ritonavir-boosted lopinavir	III, B
Sofosbuvir-based regimens should not be used with tipranavir	III, B
Ribavirin should not be used with didanosine, stavudine, or zidovudine	III, B

Patients with HIV/HCV coinfection. Hepatitis C guidance: AASLD-IDSA recommendations for testing, managing, and treating adults infected with HCV.

From American Association for the Study of Liver Diseases/ Infectious Diseases Society of America HCV Guidance Panel. Patients with HIV/HCV coinfection. Hepatitis C guidance: AASLD-IDSA recommendations for testing, managing, and treating adults infected with hepatitis C virus Web site. Available at: https://www.hcvguidelines.org/unique-populations/hiv-hcv. Published 2019. Accessed December 22, 2019. With permission.

monitor for adverse events, and screen for drug-drug interactions.[24] Individuals with type 2 diabetes as well as individuals on anticoagulation therapy require special counseling and monitoring. Individuals with type 2 diabetes must be educated on the risks of hypoglycemia associated with DAAs.[24] Patients on anticoagulation therapy should have INRs closely monitored for subtherapeutic values.[24]

Throughout treatment, it is important to closely monitor liver function to assess for worsening liver disease. DAA therapy should be discontinued if there is a 10-fold increase in ALT, especially when there is an increase in levels of other liver function markers such as conjugated bilirubin, ALP, or INR. Patients should be assessed for symptoms of worsening liver function during physical examination.[24]

Table 5
Recommendation for patients with chronic kidney disease stages 4 or 5

Recommended	Rating
No dose adjustment in DAAs is required when using recommended regimens[a]	I, A or IIa, B[b]

CKD stages: 1 = normal (estimated glomerular filtration rate [eGFR] >90 mL/min); 2 = mild CKD (eGFR 60–89 mL/min); 3 = moderate CKD (eGFR 30–59 mL/min); 4 = severe CKD (eGFR 15–29 mL/min); 5 = end-stage CKD (eGFR<15 mL/min).

[a] A ribavirin dose reduction may be required for patients with CKD stage 3, 4, or 5; see prescribing information for details.

[b] The rating is I, A for patients with CKD stage 1, 2, or 3 and IIa, B for those with CKD stage 4 or 5.

From American Association for the Study of Liver Diseases/ Infectious Diseases Society of America HCV Guidance Panel. Patients with Renal Impairment. Available at: https://www.hcvguidelines.org/unique-populations/renal-impairment. Last Update: December 2019. With permission.

After completing 12 weeks or more of therapy, a quantitative HCV viral load should be checked to confirm cure SVR.[32] When cure SVR is achieved, patients have the same follow-up recommendations as those that never had HCV.[32] If liver tests persistently remain abnormal after cure SVR is achieved, it is recommended that causes other than HCV be considered.[32] Testing for HCV recurrence is only recommended if liver function tests remain abnormal and other causes of hepatic impairment have been ruled out or the patient has sustained risk factors for HCV exposure.[32] If cure SVR is not achieved, retreatment should be considered using the guidelines discussed earlier for treatment-experienced patients.[32] Although it is not recommended that monitoring for HCV drug resistance-associated substitutions (RASs) be performed during or after treatment, it is recommended that RAS testing be completed for initiating retreatment.[24]

SUMMARY

HCV is a common blood-borne infection that can manifest in acute and chronic phases. With rates of HCV infection increasing in the United States and worldwide, the development of new DAAs has changed the way HCV can be treated. Although HCV once was a viral infection with no treatment, it can now be treated and cured. Primary care providers need to be aware of the risk factors (most notably injected drug use), pathophysiology, and appropriate diagnostic testing. Although no vaccine for HCV exists, treatment with DAAs is curative and can decrease the incidence of this viral disease.

REFERENCES

1. U.S. Preventive Services Task Force. Final recommendation statement: Hepatitis C: Screening. 2019. Available at: https://www.uspreventiveservicestaskforce.org/Page/Document/RecommendationStatementFinal/hepatitis-c-screening. Accessed December 12, 2019.
2. World Health Organization. Hepatitis C. Fact sheets Web site. 2019. Available at: https://www.who.int/news-room/fact-sheets/detail/hepatitis-c. Accessed December 13, 2020.
3. Centers for Disease Control and Prevention. Hepatitis C questions and answers for health professionals. 2020. Available at: https://www.cdc.gov/hepatitis/hcv/hcvfaq.htm. Accessed January 4, 2020.
4. American Association for the Study of Liver Diseases/Infectious Diseases Society of America HCV Guidance Panel. HCV testing and linkage to care. Hepatitis C guidance: AASLD-IDSA recommendations for testing, managing, and treating adults infected with hepatitis C virus Web site. 2019. Available at: https://www.hcvguidelines.org/evaluate/testing-and-linkage. Accessed December 1, 2019.
5. Goossens N, Clément S, Negro F. Introduction. In: Goossens N, Clément S, Negro F, editors. Handbook of hepatitis C. Cham (Switzerland): Springer International Publishing; 2016. p. 1–11.
6. Alter HJ, Purcell RH, Shih JW, et al. Detection of antibody to hepatitis C virus in prospectively followed transfusion recipients with acute and chronic non-A, non-B hepatitis. N Engl J Med 1989;321(22):1494–500.
7. Wedemeyer H. Hepatitis C. In: Feldman M, Friedman LS, Brandt LJ, editors. Sleisenger and Fordtran's gastrointestinal and liver disease. 10th edition. Philadelphia: Saunders/Elsevier; 2016. p. 1332–51.
8. Webster DP, Klenerman P, Dusheiko GM. Hepatitis C. Lancet 2015;385(9973): 1124–35.

9. Mikolajczyk AE, Te HS. Epidemiology of Hepatitis C. In: Reau N, Jensen DM, editors. The new hepatitis C: effective clinical management in the age of all-oral therapy. 2nd edition. New York: Oxford University Press; 2018. p. 7–16.

10. Han Q, Fan X, Wang X, et al. High sustained virologic response rates of sofosbuvir-based regimens in Chinese patients with HCV genotype 3a infection in a real-world setting. Virol J 2019;16(1):74.

11. Wandeler G, Dufour J-F, Bruggmann P, et al. Hepatitis C: a changing epidemic. Swiss Med Wkly 2015;145:w14093.

12. Benova L, Mohamoud YA, Calvert C, et al. Vertical transmission of hepatitis C virus: Systematic review and meta-analysis. Clin Infect Dis 2014;59(6):765–73.

13. Lockart I, Matthews GV, Danta M. Sexually transmitted hepatitis C infection: the evolving epidemic in HIV-positive and HIV-negative MSM. Curr Opin Infect Dis 2019;32(1):31–7.

14. Bartenschlager R, Lohmann V, Penin F. The molecular and structural basis of advanced antiviral therapy for hepatitis C virus infection. Nat Rev Microbiol 2013;11(7):482–96.

15. Dustin LB, Bartolini B, Capobianchi MR, et al. Hepatitis C virus: life cycle in cells, infection and host response, and analysis of molecular markers influencing the outcome of infection and response to therapy. Clin Microbiol Infect 2016; 22(10):826–32.

16. Manns MP, Buti M, Gane E, et al. Hepatitis C virus infection. Nat Rev Dis Primers 2017;3:17006.

17. Pawlotsky J-M. Pathophysiology of hepatitis C virus infection and related liver disease. Trends Microbiol 2004;12(2):96–102.

18. Goodman ZD, Makhlouf HR, Liu L, et al. Pathology of chronic hepatitis C in children: Liver biopsy findings in the Peds-C Trial. Hepatology 2008;47(3):836–43.

19. Bandiera S, Bian CB, Hoshida Y, et al. Chronic hepatitis C virus infection and pathogenesis of hepatocellular carcinoma. Curr Opin Virol 2016;20:99–105.

20. Drobnik A, Judd C, Banach D, et al. Public health implications of rapid hepatitis C screening with an oral swab for community-based organizations serving high-risk populations. Am J Public Health 2011;101(11):2151–5.

21. Collier MG, Holtzman D, Holmberg SD. Hepatitis C virus. In: Long SS, Prober CG, Fischer M, editors. Principles and practice of pediatric infectious diseases. Fifth Edition. Philadelphia: Elsevier; 2018. p. 1135–42.e3.

22. American Association for the Study of Liver Diseases/Infectious Diseases Society of America HCV Guidance Panel. Initial treatment of adults with HCV infection. Hepatitis C guidance: AASLD-IDSA recommendations for testing, managing, and treating adults infected with hepatitis C virus Web site. 2019. Available at: https://www.hcvguidelines.org/treatment-naive. Accessed November 22, 2019.

23. American Association for the Study of Liver Diseases/Infectious Diseases Society of America HCV Guidance Panel. Introduction. Hepatitis C guidance: AASLD-IDSA recommendations for testing, managing, and treating adults infected with hepatitis C virus Web site. 2019. Available at: https://www.hcvguidelines.org/contents/welcome. Accessed November 19, 2019.

24. American Association for the Study of Liver Diseases/Infectious Diseases Society of America HCV Guidance Panel. Simplified HCV treatment for treatment-naive patients without cirrhosis. Hepatitis C guidance: AASLD-IDSA recommendations for testing, managing, and treating adults infected with hepatitis C virus Web site. 2019. Available at: https://www.hcvguidelines.org/treatment-naive/simplified-treatment. Accessed December 12, 2019.

25. American Association for the Study of Liver Diseases/Infectious Diseases Society of America HCV Guidance Panel. Retreatment of persons in whom prior therapy failed. Hepatitis C guidance: AASLD-IDSA recommendations for testing, managing, and treating adults infected with hepatitis C virus Web site. 2019. Available at: https://www.hcvguidelines.org/Treatment-Experienced. Accessed November 25, 2019.

26. Ayoub WS, Tran TT. Regimens for the hepatitis C treatment-naive patient. Clin Liver Dis 2015;19(4):619–27.

27. American Association for the Study of Liver Diseases/Infectious Diseases Society of America HCV Guidance Panel. Patients with decompensated cirrhosis. Hepatitis C guidance: AASLD-IDSA recommendations for testing, managing, and treating adults infected with hepatitis C virus Web site. 2019. Available at: https://www.hcvguidelines.org/unique-populations/decompensated-cirrhosis. Accessed January 7, 2019.

28. American Association for the Study of Liver Diseases/Infectious Diseases Society of America HCV Guidance Panel. Patients with HIV/HCV coinfection. Hepatitis C guidance: AASLD-IDSA recommendations for testing, managing, and treating adults infected with hepatitis C virus Web site. 2019. Available at: https://www.hcvguidelines.org/unique-populations/hiv-hcv. Accessed December 22, 2019.

29. De Monte A, Courjon J, Anty R, et al. Direct-acting antiviral treatment in adults infected with hepatitis C virus: Reactivation of hepatitis B virus coinfection as a further challenge. J Clin Virol 2016;78:27–30.

30. American Association for the Study of Liver Diseases/Infectious Diseases Society of America HCV Guidance Panel. Patients with renal impairment. Hepatitis C guidance: AASLD-IDSA recommendations for testing, managing, and treating adults infected with hepatitis C virus Web site. 2019. Available at: https://www.hcvguidelines.org/unique-populations/renal-impairment. Accessed January 9, 2019.

31. Coppola N, De Pascalis S, Pisaturo M, et al. Sustained virological response to antiviral treatment in chronic hepatitis C patients may be predictable by HCV-RNA clearance in peripheral blood mononuclear cells. J Clin Virol 2013;58(4): 748–50.

32. American Association for the Study of Liver Diseases/Infectious Diseases Society of America HCV Guidance Panel. Monitoring patients who are starting HCV treatment, are on treatment, or have completed therapy. Hepatitis C guidance: AASLD-IDSA recommendations for testing, managing, and treating adults infected with hepatitis C virus Web site. 2019. Available at: https://www.hcvguidelines.org/evaluate/monitoring. Accessed January 8, 2020.

The Reemergence of Syphilis
Clinical Pearls for Consideration

Mary McNamara, DNP, FNP-BC[a],*, Charles Yingling, DNP, FNP-BC[b]

KEYWORDS

- Syphilis • STI • Epidemiology • Men who have sex with men (MSM)

KEY POINTS

- Although nearly eradicated in the United States by 1998, syphilis incidence rates have been increasing since 2000.
- Rates of congenital syphilis and syphilitic stillbirths have increased significantly in the past 5 years.
- Syphilis disproportionately affects people of color, men who have sex with men, and transgender women.
- Syphilis is the "great imitator" and nurses should consider a diagnosis of syphilis in people with classic and less common symptoms.

INTRODUCTION

Although nearly eradicated in the United States by 1998, syphilis incidence rates have been increasing since 2000.[1] Nurses, positioned throughout the health care system, are equipped to screen for, diagnose, and treat syphilis in its primary, secondary, and tertiary stages. This article describes the history of syphilis, reviews current guidelines for diagnosis and treatment, and introduces strategies for reducing rates of new syphilis infections.

HISTORY

Syphilis is known as the "great imitator" due to varied clinical presentations and the potential time interval between infection and symptom onset. Syphilis is the oldest known sexually transmitted infection (STI).[2] *Treponema pallidum* was identified as the causative bacterium for syphilis by Fritz Schaudinn and Erich Hoffmann in Germany in 1905, and the first diagnostic test for the infection was invented in 1906.[2]

[a] Department of Population Health Nursing Science, University of Illinois at Chicago College of Nursing, Chicago, IL, USA; [b] Department of Population Health Nursing Science, University of Illinois at Chicago College of Nursing, 845 South Damen Avenue, Chicago, IL 60612, USA
* Corresponding author. UIC College of Nursing, 1601 Parkview, S-313, Rockford, IL 61107.
E-mail address: mmcnam5@uic.edu
Twitter: @marymackaprn (M.M.); @CharlieUIC (C.Y.)

Nurs Clin N Am 55 (2020) 361–377
https://doi.org/10.1016/j.cnur.2020.06.009
0029-6465/20/© 2020 Elsevier Inc. All rights reserved.

Initially treated with highly toxic and ineffective mercury and arsphenamine,[3] in 1943, John Mahoney introduced penicillin, revolutionizing the treatment of syphilis.[3] Penicillin remains the mainstay of syphilis treatment nearly 80 years after its introduction.

Development of diagnostic and treatment guidelines has been fraught with ethical lapses, including the inhumane treatment of human subjects.[4-10] In 1837, a French-American physician, Philippe Ricord, demonstrated that gonorrhea and syphilis were distinct STIs by injecting 17 prisoners in Parisian jails.[2] Ricord also is credited as the first to describe the primary, secondary, and latent stages of syphilis. The US Public Health Service did similarly inoculate 1300 Guatemalan sex workers, prisoners, mental health patients, and soldiers with syphilis and gonorrhea from 1946 to 1948 while treating just more than half of those human subjects.[6,7] The infamous "ethically impossible"[8] Tuskegee Syphilis Study also notoriously and knowingly withheld penicillin treatment from hundreds of primarily rural and poor Black American men infected with syphilis for 40 years (1932–1972).[8,9] These experiments accelerated health disparities while decreasing health care utilization and health-seeking behaviors among populations that continue to have a disproportionately high incidence of multiple health problems, including syphilis.[10]

MICROBIOLOGY

T pallidum, the syphilis spirochete, is deemed the "stealth pathogen."[11] Adept at dissemination and immune evasion, syphilis infection can lead to chronic latent and tertiary infection.[11] Left untreated, syphilis infection can span decades. Despite being the oldest and earliest discovered STI, understanding of syphilis has not kept pace with knowledge of other bacterial infections. Pathogenic species of treponemes defy study due to being slow growing, poorly tolerant of desiccation and temperature extremes, and nearly unculturable.[11,12] Despite *T pallidum* being one of the first bacterial genomes to be sequenced, its pathogenesis, virulence, and gene expression are still incompletely understood.[12,13]

Spirochetes can deftly penetrate mucous membranes or breaks in skin barrier from sexual activity. Their morphology propels their dissemination. They lack surface-exposed lipoproteins that activate macrophages and dendritic cells, allowing evasion from destruction by the immune system.[12] *T pallidum* is the most virulent *Treponema* subspecies and easily crosses the blood-brain barrier and the maternal-fetal placenta.[11]

CLINICAL PRESENTATION

Recognition of primary and secondary (P&S) syphilis is crucial to decreasing disease transmission. Syphilis should be included in the differential diagnosis of any sexually active person with a rash or genital lesion. A solitary, painless, indurated genital chancre (ulcer) smaller than 2 cm is the hallmark of primary syphilis infection.[1,14-16] The chancre heals spontaneously in approximately 3 weeks to 4 weeks and is 98% specific and 31% sensitive in identifying primary infection.[17] Clinical findings of secondary syphilis may include fever, swollen glands, patchy hair loss, condyloma lata, oral or perineal gray or white patches, and other skin rashes.[1,14] The rash associated with secondary syphilis usually is nonpruritic and symmetrically distributed and may involve the palms and soles.

After the P&S stages of syphilis, patients progress to either latent or tertiary syphilis. Latent syphilis is defined as either early or late and based on the interval since initial infection. Early latent syphilis occurs within 12 months of exposure. Late latent syphilis can be defined as either greater than 1 year since initial infection or unknown time since exposure. Tertiary syphilis may occur 1 year to decades after initial infection.

Tertiary syphilis may be characterized as gummatous, cardiovascular, and/or neurologic.[1,14] Gummata are noncancerourous granulomatous lesions found in multiple tissues, including the brain, liver, testes, bone, and skin. Cardiovascular complications of tertiary syphilis can include valve disorders and aortic aneurysm.[1,14] Central nervous system infection can occur at any stage. Early neurosyphilis findings include hearing and vision changes, meningitis, and altered mental status.[18] Tabes dorsalis occurs 10 years to 30 years after primary infection and is the result of an untreated syphilis infection that slowly degenerates nerve tissue, resulting in weakness, diminished reflexes, unsteady gait, joint pain, loss of coordination, paralysis, personality changes, dementia, deafness, visual impairment, and impaired pupillary reaction to light.[18] **Fig. 1** and **Table 1** describes the stages of syphilis. Symptoms correlate with stages and infection transmission.

DIAGNOSIS AND TREATMENT

The threshold for serologic testing should be low. The US Preventive Services Task Force (USPSTF) recommends routine screening in adolescents and adults at high risk,[19] defined as men who have sex with men (MSM) and individuals with human immunodeficiency virus (HIV).[1] Risk factors dependent on prevalence include men under age 29, sex work, drug use, and history of incarceration within the past 12 months.[1] Testing should be offered to anyone with increased risk factors or signs and symptoms of P&S infection.

Because of antepartum fetal infection and congenital syphilis (CS), all pregnant women require screening. The USPSTF[20] and the Centers for Disease Control and Prevention (CDC)[1] recommend screening all pregnant women at their first prenatal visit. Multiple state laws mandate screening at the first prenatal visit and in the third trimester.[21]

Syphilis must be diagnosed with serologic testing because T pallidum is difficult to culture. Diagnosis is based on treponemal (fluorescent treponemal antibody absorption [FTA-ABS], enzyme-linked immunoassays [EIAs], and treponemal pallidum particle agglutination [TP-PA]) and nontreponemal (Venereal Disease Research Laboratory [VDRL] and rapid plasma reagin [RPR]) serologic testing, as shown in **Table 2**. Treponemal tests detect antibodies to T pallidum proteins. Nontreponemal tests detect antibodies to damaged host cells and lipoidal antigens.[22] Nontreponemal serology historically has been the standard, initial, cost-effective screening in the United States and still is recommended by the CDC. Reactive RPR results are recorded as quantitative titers. RPR may remain nonreactive, however, for up to 4 weeks after initial infection and often is negative in primary syphilis.[23] A negative RPR, in the absence of treatment, 3 months after potential exposure, rules out syphilis infection.[1,23] Traditionally, treponemal testing is used to confirm reactive nontreponemal results.[23,24] Reverse sequence screening, or initially testing with treponemal and confirmed by nontreponemal serology, has gained favor due to immunoassay automation. Inconclusive results should be verified, as demonstrated in **Table 3**. Patients with syphilis should be screened routinely for chlamydia, gonorrhea, and HIV.[1,23,25] Further testing is warranted for persons with clinical signs of neurosyphilis or tabes dorsalis.[25–27] A diagnosis of neurosyphilis depends on a combination of neurologic symptoms, reactive serology tests, and cerebrospinal fluid (CSF) tests, including CSF cell count, CSF protein, and a reactive CSF-VDRL.[1,27] In both the United States and Canada, all jurisdictions require reporting of new syphilis diagnoses to public health authorities.

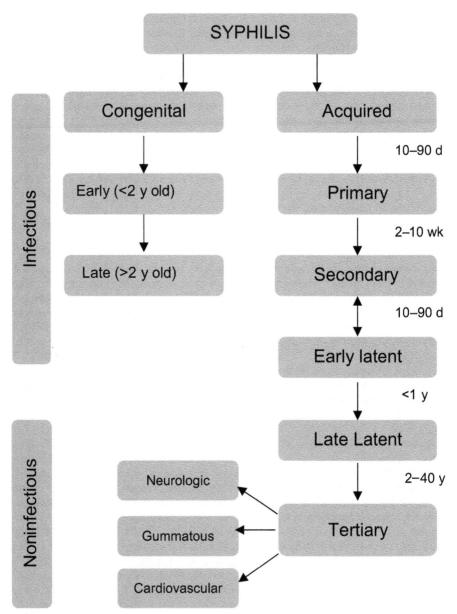

Fig. 1. Stages of syphilis. (*Data from* Centers for Disease Control and Prevention. Sexually Transmitted Disease Surveillance 2018. Atlanta: U.S. Department of Health and Human Services; 2019. Available at: https://www.cdc.gov/std/stats18/STDSurveillance2018-full-report. pdf; and From Centers for Disease Control and Prevention. Sexually Transmitted Diseases: Syphilis – CDC Fact Sheet. Available at: https://www.cdc.gov/std/syphilis/stdfact-syphilis. htm; with permission; and Aguinaldo J. TORCH(Z) Congenital Infections. St. George's University, Masters of Public Health Program. Available at: http://mph.sgu.edu/mphblog/2017/05/ 16/torchz-congenital-infections/; with permission.)

Table 1
Stages of syphilis

Primary stage	Onset 10–90 d postexposure Duration 3–6 wk	Single chancre; usually firm, round, and painless; <2 cm; and located where *T pallidum* enters the body	
Secondary stage	Onset 4–10 wk after primary Duration varies, usually 2 mo	Rash of multiple locations and morphologies, especially palms of hands and soles of feet; fever; swollen nodes; sore throat; patchy hair loss; headaches and neurologic changes; weight loss; myalgias; fatigue	
Latent stage	Onset at end of secondary stage Duration 1–20 y	Asymptomatic May experience multiple relapses of secondary syphilis before returning to latent stage	

(continued on next page)

Table 1
(continued)

Tertiary stage	May occur at any point or never occur	Dependent on affected organs Gummata, cardiovascular, ocular syphilis, neurosyphilis Tabes dorsalis	
Congenital	Contracted through placenta or during labor and delivery	Saddle nose, Hutchinson teeth, interstitial keratitis, deafness, skeletal deformities, neurosyphilis	

Data from Centers for Disease Control and Prevention. Sexually Transmitted Disease Surveillance 2018. Atlanta: U.S. Department of Health and Human Services; 2019.

Table 2
Diagnostic testing for syphilis

Nontreponemal serologic	VDRL or RPR	Considerations
Treponemal serologic	FTA-ABS tests TP-PA assay EIAs, CLIAs , immunoblots, or rapid treponemal assays	Use of only 1 type of serologic test is insufficient for diagnosis and can result in false-negative and false-positive results. Nontreponemal test should be done first, and, if reactive, must be followed by treponemal testing to confirm diagnosis. Follow-up with RPR to track response to treatment and disease activity. Few treponemal tests are approved for use in the United States.
Direct detection: PCR, dark-field microscopy, direct fluorescent antibody	Not widely commercially available	Definitive diagnosis

Data from CDC Sexually Transmitted Infection Treatment Guidelines 2015. Diagnostic Considerations And CDC Discordant results from reverse sequence syphilis screening–five laboratories, United States, 2006-2010.

Parenteral penicillin G is the preferred treatment of all individuals and all stages of syphilis.[28] Parenteral penicillin G is the only acceptable therapy for syphilis during pregnancy.[28] Pregnant women who report penicillin allergy should be desensitized and treated with penicillin.[28,29] The duration and preparation of penicillin G treatment depend on syphilis stage and clinical manifestations, as shown in **Table 4**. Penicillin G benzathine, 2.4 million U, injected intramuscularly (IM) in a single dose, appropriately treats adults with P&S and early latent syphilis. Treatment with penicillin G procaine is not appropriate and should be carefully avoided. Infants and children with P&S syphilis should receive penicillin G benzathine, 50,000 U/kg IM, up to the adult dose of 2.4 million U, in a single dose. Treat late latent and tertiary syphilis with penicillin G benzathine, 2.4 million U IM weekly for 3 weeks. Neurosyphilis is treated with aqueous crystalline penicillin G, 18 million U to 24 million U, intravenously, daily for 10 days

Table 3
Inconclusive diagnostic testing for syphilis

Test Results	Conclusion
Positive reactive RPR with negative EIA/CLIA and TP-PA	False-positive RPR
Positive EIA/CLIA with negative confirmatory TP-PA and negative RPR	False-positive vs early infection
Positive EIA/CLIA with indeterminant confirmatory TP-PA and negative RPR	New infection vs waning antibodies from previous treated infection

Data from CDC Sexually Transmitted Infection Treatment Guidelines 2015. Diagnostic Considerations And CDC Discordant results from reverse sequence syphilis screening–five laboratories, United States, 2006-2010.

Table 4
Syphilis treatment guidelines in immunocompetent people

Stage	First Line	Alternate	Considerations
Primary, secondary, and early latent	Penicillin G benzathine, 2.4 million U IM once	Tetracycline, 500 mg PO QID for 14 d OR Doxycycline, 100 mg PO BID for 14 d	6-mo and 12-mo serologic and clinical evaluation HIV testing at diagnosis and at 3 mo in areas of high prevalence
Latent >1 y	Penicillin G benzathine, 2.4 million U IM weekly for 3 wk	Tetracycline 500 mg PO QID for 28 d OR Doxycycline, 100 mg PO BID for 28 d	Consider ophthalmic and CSF evaluation if neurologic symptoms present 6-mo and 12-mo serologic and clinical evaluation HIV testing at diagnosis in all patients
Tertiary	Penicillin G benzathine, 2.4 million U IM weekly for 3 wk	Tetracycline, 500 mg PO QID for 28 d OR Doxycycline, 100 mg PO BID for 28 d	
Pregnancy	Parenteral penicillin G benzathine per corresponding stage of infection	No appropriate alternative Attempt to desensitize penicillin allergy	Treatment must be 30 d prior to delivery. Serologic titers at 28–32 wk gestation and at delivery
Contacts	Penicillin G benzathine, 2.4 million U IM	Tetracycline, 500 mg PO QID for 14 d OR Doxycycline, 100 mg PO BID for 14 d	Provide nonjudgmental help contacting partners confidentially, to reduce reinfection and transmission

Contacts have had sex with person with early syphilis within 90 d.
Data from CDC Sexually Transmitted Infection Treatment Guidelines 2015.

to 14 days. Individuals receiving treatment, especially in P&S stages, should be informed that they may experience Jarisch-Herxheimer reaction, including fever, myalgias, and headache, in the first 24 hours of treatment. Comprehensive treatment guidelines are available from the CDC.[28]

EPIDEMIOLOGY

Rates of once-rare syphilis are increasing globally, especially affecting Black men, HIV-positive people, and MSM.[1] In 2018, 115,045 total cases of all stages of syphilis were reported in the United States, the highest number of total cases since 1991.[1] This represents a 13.3% increase from 2017 (101,584 cases). Since nearly eradicated at the end of the 1990s, syphilis incidence continues to increase across ethnic groups (**Tables 5 and 6**; see **Table 8**), age and sex (**Fig. 2**), and geographic regions (**Tables 7 and 8**). **Fig. 3** shows the distribution of total P&S cases in 2018. The greatest percent increases from 2017 to 2018 have occurred in men ages 20 to 34, Black men, MSM, and people who use drugs. Incidence in all women and women of childbearing age, however, also has increased (172.7% and 165.4%, respectively) from 2014 to 2018.[1]

CS rates have paralleled the increases observed in women. CS rates in the United States have risen 153% since 2013 (9.2 cases per 100,000 live births), which was the first increase since 2008. Seventy percent of CS cases were reported from just 5 states (Texas, Florida, California, Arizona, and Louisiana), but most states reported

Table 5
Comparing rates of primary and secondary syphilis the United States by ethnicity, 1998 versus 2018

Race/Ethnicity	1998	2018
American Indians/Alaskan Natives	2.8	15.5
Blacks	17.1	28.1
Hispanics	1.5	13
Whites	0.5	6.0
Asians	0.4	4.6

[a] Rate per 100,000 population.
Data from Centers for Disease Control and Prevention. Sexually Transmitted Disease Surveillance 2018. Atlanta: U.S. Department of Health and Human Services; 2019.

at least 1 case of CS in 2018.[1] The United States 2018 CS rate (33.1 cases per 100,000 live births) represents a 39.7% increase from to 2017 and a 185.3% increase from 2014 (**Table 9**). Syphilitic stillbirths also have increased from 63 in 2017 to 78 in 2018. There was a 22% increase in newborn deaths from syphilis from 77 in 2017 to 94 in 2018.

Drivers of the Epidemic

Multiple determinants drive these trends. These determinants include but are not limited to health-seeking behaviors, access to care, risk-taking behaviors, and provider education and training.[10,30,31] Health-seeking behaviors are limited partly by lack of trust in the health care system,[10] limited awareness about syphilis risk,[1] and the belief that syphilis is a disease of antiquity.[1,2] Access to care is impeded in part by poverty, stigma, lack of transportation, and unstable housing.[1,10,30,31] Reduced access also results from the high cost of care and inadequate or no insurance coverage. Healthy People 2020 cites the lack of availability of services as a limiting factor for access.[31] Health inequity contributes to a higher syphilis incidence and prevalence in ethnic and sexual minority groups (see **Table 8**).

Lack of access has been further exacerbated by budget cuts, including Title X federal grants that fund reproductive health services in the United States.[32,33] The domestic gag rule, instituted in 2019 and applied to clinics receiving Title X funding, prohibits the provision of or referral to abortion services. This rule impacted more than 900 women's health clinics nationwide, including health departments, federally

Table 6
Increasing rates of primary and secondary syphilis in the United States by ethnicity from 2017 to 2018

Race/Ethnicity	Increase (%)
American Indian/Alaskan Natives	40.9
Multiracial	22.1
Native Hawaiians/Pacific Islanders	19.0
Blacks	17.1
Hispanics	13.0
Whites	11.1

Data from Centers for Disease Control and Prevention. Sexually Transmitted Disease Surveillance 2018. Atlanta: U.S. Department of Health and Human Services; 2019.

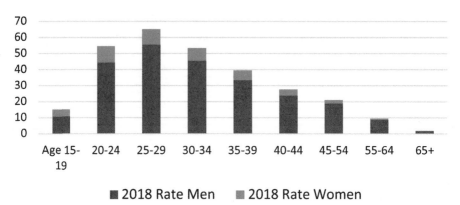

Fig. 2. US rate of cases of P&S syphilis by age and sex, 2018. Rate per 100,000 population. (*Data from* Centers for Disease Control and Prevention. Sexually Transmitted Disease Surveillance 2018. Atlanta: U.S. Department of Health and Human Services; 2019. Available at: https://www.cdc.gov/std/stats18/STDSurveillance2018-full-report.pdf.)

qualified health centers, and other nonprofit providers. Latinas account for one-third and women of color account for more than half of patients served in Title X sites. Twenty-three percent of Title X sites have declared that they will not use Title X funds as result of this rule, having an impact on early prenatal care and screening for P&S syphilis and CS. Budget cuts have made it difficult for clinics to offer free STI screening and treatment.[1,32,33]

Risk-taking behaviors, such as decreased or incorrect condom use, are fueled by drug use,[34–36] technology,[37] and age.[1,38] People who use drugs report higher-risk sexual behaviors, including multiple partners and lack of condom use. Drug use has more than doubled among heterosexual people with P&S syphilis from 2013 to 2017.[25] Although the greatest proportion of P&S syphilis occurs in MSM, sexually disinhibiting drug use increased most in women and heterosexual men (men who have sex with women [MSW]) with P&S syphilis, and included injection drug use, methamphetamine use, heroin use, and sex with people who inject drugs.[25] Although the number of MSM cases reporting injection drug use, methamphetamine use, and heroin use increased slightly, the proportion of MSM with P&S cases reporting use of these drugs did not. Injection drug use by women increased from 4.0% in 2013% to 10.5% in 2017, and MSW cases reporting injection drug use increased from 2.8% to 6.3%. By region, injection drug use was highest in the West and lowest in the Northeast. Injection drug use was most prevalent among Alaskan Natives/American Indians and whites.

Table 7
Comparing rates (per 100,000 population) of primary and secondary syphilis by US geographic region, 1998 versus 2018

Region	1998	2018
South	5.1	7.1
West	1.0	15.0
Midwest	1.5	13
Northeast	0.8	8.7

Data from Centers for Disease Control and Prevention. *Sexually Transmitted Disease Surveillance 2018.* Atlanta: U.S. Department of Health and Human Services; 2019.

Table 8
Rate increase of primary and secondary syphilis, 2017 to 2018, by region and ethnicity

	Rate Increase, 2017–2018 (%)
By US geographic region	
South	15.6
West	15.4
Midwest	16.4
Northeast	10.1
By ethnicity	
Black	17.1
Multiple	22.1
American Indian	40.9
Native Hawaiian	19.1
White	11.1
Asian	9.5

Data from Centers for Disease Control and Prevention. Sexually Transmitted Disease Surveillance 2018. Atlanta: U.S. Department of Health and Human Services; 2019.

Methamphetamine use in women with P&S syphilis increased from 6.2% to 16.6% from 2013 to 2017. Methamphetamine use among MSW affected by P&S syphilis increased from 5.0% to 13.3%. The proportion of MSM with P&S syphilis cases reporting methamphetamine use decreased from 9.2% to 8.0%. The proportion of P&S syphilis cases that used heroin more than doubled among female cases and more than tripled among MSW cases but remained stable among MSM cases.[25]

Increased risk-taking behaviors also may be attributable to increased technology and dating apps.[37] With the rise of dating and hookup apps, such as Grindr, Tinder, and Scruff, it is not only easier to meet anonymous sex partners but also more difficult to track them down to facilitate partner treatment.

Risk-taking behaviors are historically higher in youth and adolescents; 15-year-old to 24-year-old individuals account for more than half of all new STIs in the United States but represent only one-quarter of the entire population.[1] In 2018, the rate of P&S syphilis among 15-year-old to 24-year-old women was 7.2 cases per 100,000

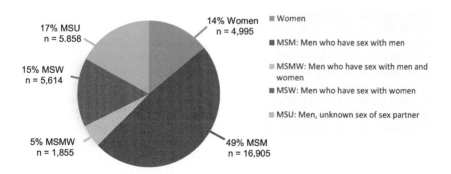

Fig. 3. Distribution of cases of P&S syphilis, 2018. (*Data from* Centers for Disease Control and Prevention. Sexually Transmitted Disease Surveillance 2018. Atlanta: U.S. Department of Health and Human Services; 2019. Available at: https://www.cdc.gov/std/stats18/STDSurveillance2018-full-report.pdf.)

Table 9
Congenital syphilis in the United States

Group	Rate 2014	Rate 2018	Percentage increase 2014-2018
CS total	11.4	33.1	185.5
CS black	38.2	86.6	126.7
CS Hispanic	12.2	44.7	266.9
CS white	3.7	13.5	264.8

[a] Rate per 100,000 live births.
Data from Centers for Disease Control and Prevention. Sexually Transmitted Disease Surveillance 2018. Atlanta: U.S. Department of Health and Human Services; 2019.

women, a 28.6% increase from 2017 (5.6 cases per 100,000 women) and a 100.0% increase from 2014 (3.6 cases per 100,000 women). Among 15-year-old to 24-year-old male cases in 2018, the rate was 28.2 cases per 100,000, a 7.2% increase from 2017 (26.3 per 100,000 male cases) and a 44.6% increase from 2014 (19.5 per 100,000 male cases).[1] These high rates may be attributed to both increased screening efforts and increased incidence.

Education and training of both the health care providers and the public are important factors in the syphilis epidemic. One in 3 providers has not received further training on STIs after graduation.[1,25] Sexual education in schools is limited and at times nonexistent and also may contribute to the epidemic.[38] Only 24 states mandate sex education. The California Healthy Youth Act went into effect in 2016 and is the most comprehensive sex education legislation in the United States. It includes education specific to students who identify as lesbian, gay, bisexual, transgender, or queer. The Act requires sexual education in seventh grade and in high school and mandates education on consent and harassment. The law has been met with resistance from conservative groups. Critics maintain that the content is not age appropriate. Similar protests challenge progressive sex education legislation in several states.[38]

Syphilis Among Men Who Have Sex with Men and Transgender Women

The diverse population of MSM is disproportionately affected with syphilis and coinfection with HIV.[1,25,39] Gay and bisexual men and transgender women who have sex with men are impacted biologically with increased susceptibility of rectal and oral mucosa to infection transmission, behaviorally in some instances due to frequent partner changes, and structurally due to stigma, bigotry, and lack of culturally competent care.[40]

Some have proposed that HIV pre-exposure prophylaxis (PrEP) has contributed to the increased syphilis incidence[41] because it may afford false security in STI prevention, increase higher-risk sexual behavior, and decrease condom use.[42,43] A 2016 meta-analysis showed that rates of new diagnoses among MSM using PrEP were 44.6-times greater for syphilis, 25.3 times greater for gonorrhea, and 11.2-times greater for chlamydia compared with MSM not taking PrEP.[43] The PROUD randomized control trial, however, strongly supported the efficacy of PrEP in preventing HIV-1, without noting new cases of other STIs.[44] It is important to consider that syphilis incidence has been rising since 2001, well before PrEP was approved by the Food and Drug Administration in 2012. PrEP adoption has been slow in locations and populations with concerning epidemiology. Syphilis incidence is increasing significantly in young adult MSM, people in the South, and in Native American individuals, all groups who have been less likely to utilize PrEP.[1,39,41] It is certain that P&S syphilis facilitates HIV transmission because sores or breaks in the skin allow the virus to enter the body more easily.[39,40] Despite the possibility of risk compensation, the benefits of HIV PrEP outweigh any possible risk of increase in syphilis infection.

STRATEGIES TO DECREASE THE TREND

Identifying and staging syphilis properly are key to appropriate treatment planning and follow-up. Syphilis may be difficult to diagnose, but it is easy to treat. Penicillin remains the most effective treatment, despite a concerning increase in penicillin resistant strains of syphilis. Penicillin cannot reverse damage caused by syphilis, only eradicate the infection. Early diagnosis is key to decreasing incidence and morbidity.[1,28] Nurses should routinely collect and revise detailed patient sexual histories, including sex partners, anatomic risk of exposure, and risk factors. Interviews should be supportive, open-ended, and nonbiased. Nontreponemal screening tests should be done at least annually on sexually active MSM, including those with HIV infection or taking PrEP. Screen as frequently as every 3 months to 6 months in all individuals if there is drug use or multiple sex partners.[23,28] All individuals with an oral, anal, or vaginal sex partner who have been recently diagnosed with syphilis should be screened. Screen all pregnant women at the initial prenatal visit and in the last trimester. Ensure partner treatment to prevent reinfection.[23,28]

Serologic and clinical follow-up are essential. Nontreponemal titers should decrease 4-fold within 6 months to 12 months and ongoing elevation in titers may indicate treatment failure.[28] Indirect nontreponemal tests (RPR and VRDL) are not diagnostic without clinical and treponemal confirmation.[11,12,22]

An emerging strategy for the early detection of syphilis includes the use of reverse sequence screening and emerging technologies for direct detection of *T pallidum*. Current CDC guidelines[1] call for the initial syphilis diagnosis to be based on indirect nontreponemal testing (RPR and VDRL) followed by treponemal testing (polymerase chain reaction [PCR], TP-TA, and FTA-ABS) (**Fig. 4**). A study of 15 cases of syphilis diagnosed between January 2013 and September 2018 at a clinic in Spain, however, demonstrated that treponemal testing (chemiluminescence immunoassays [CLIAs] and EIAs) were useful in diagnosing early syphilis. Of 158 total individuals diagnosed with syphilis, 15 subjects had negative nontreponemal tests (RPR), and 14 of 15 had syphilis detected by treponemal testing in early primary syphilis. Treponemal PCR detected *T pallidum* in the primary lesion exudate of 8 subjects. The study promotes reverse sequence treponemal testing as the future of initial screening, given diagnostic sensitivity, speed, and low cost.[45] This assertion should be further evaluated as a potential strategy to reverse the current epidemiologic trend through prompt diagnosis. **Fig. 4** compares traditional screening to reverse screening. Although reverse screening algorithms (ie, treponemal testing confirmed by nontreponemal testing) recently have gained favor due to immunoassay automation, the CDC currently continues to recommend the traditional screening algorithm.

CASE EXAMPLE

A 22-year-old man in usual good health presented to his nurse practitioner with a rash that started 1 week prior to the office visit. He denied systemic symptoms and exposure to any new detergents, soaps, persons with rash, or outdoor activity. The nurse practitioner took a careful and culturally sensitive sexual history and the patient disclosed regular sexual activity with 2 male partners. The patient reported careful condom use with every sexual encounter. Nontreponemal testing (RPR) was obtained. The RPR and additional STI tests were negative. The patient was referred to dermatology and diagnosed with discoid eczema. He showed no improvement with

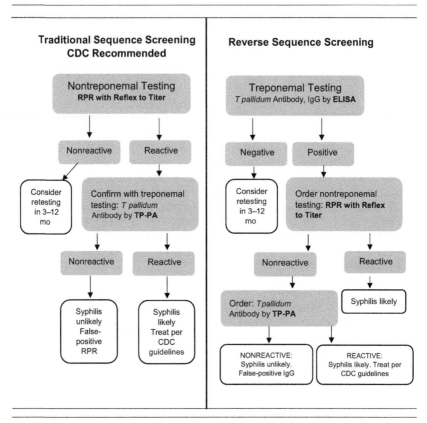

Fig. 4. Syphilis testing algorithms. (*Adapted from* ARUP Consult. Syphilis Testing Algorithms. Arup Laboratories. December 2019. Available at: https://arupconsult.com/algorithm/syphilis-testing-algorithm. With permission ©2019 ARUP Laboratories. All Rights Reserved.)

emollients and topical corticosteroids. About 6 weeks after rash onset, he reported feeling mentally "foggy." While under treatment of his rash, he hit his head during a motor vehicle collision, and subsequent diagnostic imaging of the brain was normal. Seven weeks after initial onset of his rash, the nurse practitioner repeated the RPR and it was positive. A syphilis diagnosis was confirmed with treponemal testing (FTA-ABS). The patient's symptoms of P&S syphilis resolved completely after a single dose of penicillin G benzathine, 2.4 million U IM.

SUMMARY

Nurses must be knowledgeable about and maintain a high index of suspicion for syphilis in patients with clinical signs and symptoms or asymptomatic people at risk. Nontreponemal testing often is negative in the first 4 weeks of infection.[22] So, follow-up testing is essential to identify many cases of P&S syphilis. Nurses may consider the use of a reverse screening algorithm because this may improve diagnostic accuracy in early primary syphilis.

The reemergence of syphilis threatens public health and nurses play an essential role in the screening, diagnosis, and treatment of syphilis in people at risk. Syphilis' reputation as the "great imitator" should remind practicing nurses to be vigilant and consider a diagnosis of syphilis in patients with both classic and less common symptoms of the disease.

DISCLOSURE

The authors have nothing to disclose.

REFERENCES

1. Centers for Disease Control and Prevention. Sexually transmitted disease surveillance, 2018. Atlanta (GA): Department of Health and Human Services; 2019. Available at: https://www.cdc.gov/std/stats18/default.htm.
2. Barnett R. Syphilis. Lancet 2018;391:1471.
3. Karamanou M, Kyriakis K, Tsoucalas G, et al. Hallmarks in the history of syphilis therapeutics. Infez Med 2013;21(4):314–7.
4. Vonderlehr RA, Clark T, Wenger OC, et al. Untreated syphilis in the male Negro: a comparative study of treated and untreated cases. JAMA 1936;107:856–60.
5. Olansky S, Schuman SH, Peters JJ, et al. Untreated syphilis in the male Negro: X. Twenty years of clinical observation of untreated syphilitic and presumably nonsyphilitic groups. AMA Arch Derm 1956;73(5):516–22.
6. U.S. Presidential Commission on Bioethical Issues. Moral science: protecting participants in human subjects research. Washington, DC: U.S. Presidential Commission for the Study of Bioethical Issues; 2011.
7. Reverby SM. Ethical failures and history lessons: the U.S. Public Health Service research studies in Tuskegee and Guatemala. Public Health Rev 2012;34. https://doi.org/10.1007/BF03391665.
8. U.S. Presidential Commission for the Study of Bioethical Issues. Ethically impossible: STD research in Guatemala from 1946 to 1948. Washington, DC: U.S. Presidential Commission for the Study of Bioethical Issues; 2011.
9. National Center for HIV/AIDS, Viral Hepatitis, STD, and TB Prevention, Centers for Disease Control and Prevention. US Public Health Service Syphilis Study at Tuskegee. Available at: https://www.cdc.gov/tuskegee/timeline.htm. Accessed December 22, 2015.
10. Alsan M, Wanamaker M. Tuskegee and the health of black men. National Bureau of Economic Research. Working Paper 22323, June 2016. Revised June 2017. Available at: http://nber.org/papers/w22323. Accessed October 18, 2019.
11. Radolf J, Deka R, Anand A, et al. Treponema pallidum, the syphilis spirochete: making a living as a stealth pathogen. Nat Rev Microbiol 2016;14:744–59.
12. Izard J, Renken C, Hsieh CE, et al. Cryo-electron tomography elucidates the molecular architecture of Treponema pallidum, the syphilis spirochete. J Bacteriol 2009;191:7566–80.
13. Frasier CM, Norris SJ, Weinstock GM, et al. Complete genome sequence of Treponema pallidum, the syphilis spirochete. Science 1998;281:375–88.
14. Hicks CB, Clement M. Syphilis: Epidemiology, pathophysiology, and clinical manifestations in HIV-uninfected patients. Retrieved from Up to Date website. 2019. Available at: https://www.uptodate.com/contents/syphilis-epidemiology-pathophysiology-and-clinical-manifestations-in-hiv-uninfected-patients?topicRef=7588&source=see_link. Accessed October 28, 2019.
15. Rompalo A. Syphilis in the HIV-infected patient 2019. Up to Date website Available at: https://www.uptodate.com/contents/syphilis-in-the-hiv-infected-patient?topicRef=7597&source=see_link. Accessed October 24, 2019.

16. Sabre L, Braschinsky M, Taba P. Neurosyphilis as a great imitator: a case report. BMC Res Notes 2016;9:372.
17. O'Byrne P, MacPhearson P. Syphilis. BMJ 2019;365:l4159.
18. National Institute of. Neurological Disorders and Stroke. Tabes Dorsalis information page. 2019. NINDS website Available at: https://www.ninds.nih.gov/Disorders/All-Disorders/Tabes-Dorsalis-Information-Page. Accessed October 24, 2019.
19. U.S. Preventative Services Task Force. Final Update Summary: Syphilis Infection in Nonpregnant Adults and Adolescents: Screening. 2016. Available at: https://www.uspreventiveservicestaskforce.org/Page/Document/UpdateSummaryFinal/syphilis-infection-in-nonpregnant-adults-and-adolescents. Accessed October 23, 2019.
20. U.S. Preventative Services Task Force. Final Update Summary: Syphilis Infection in Pregnant Women: Screening. 2018. Available at: https://www.uspreventiveservicestaskforce.org/Page/Document/UpdateSummaryFinal/syphilis-infection-in-pregnancy-screening1. Accessed October 23, 2019.
21. Centers for Disease Control and Prevention, Division of STD Prevention, National Center for HIV/AIDS, Viral Hepatitis, STD, and TB Prevention. State Statutory and Regulatory Language Regarding Prenatal Syphilis Screenings in the United States, 2018. 2019. Available at: https://www.cdc.gov/std/treatment/syphilis-screenings-2018.htm. Accessed October 18, 2019.
22. Henao-Martinez AF, Johnson SC. Diagnostic tests for syphilis: new tests and new algorithms. Neurol Clin Pract 2014;4(2):114–22.
23. Hicks CB, Clement M. Syphilis: screening and diagnostic testing 2019. Up to Date website Available at: https://www.uptodate.com/contents/syphilis-screening-and-diagnostic-testing. Accessed October 24, 2019.
24. Centers for Disease Control and Prevention. Discordant results from reverse sequence syphilis screening–five laboratories, United States, 2006-2010. MMWR Morb Mortal Wkly Rep 2011;60(5):133–7. Available at: https://www.cdc.gov/mmwr/preview/mmwrhtml/mm6005a1.htm.
25. Centers for Disease Control and Prevention. Syphilis surveillance supplement 2013–2017. Atlanta (GA): U.S. Department of Health and Human Services; 2019. Available at: https://www.cdc.gov/std/stats17/syphilis2017/default.htm.
26. Poliseli R, Vidal JE, Penalva De Oliveira AC, et al. Neurosyphilis in HIV-infected patients: clinical manifestations, serum venereal disease research laboratory titers, and associated factors to symptomatic neurosyphilis. Sex Transm Dis 2008;35:425.
27. Moradi A, Salek S, Daniel E, et al. Clinical features and incidence rates of ocular complications in patients with ocular syphilis. Am J Ophthalmol 2015;159:334.
28. Centers for Disease Control and Prevention. Sexually Transmitted Diseases Treatment Guidelines, 2015. MMWR Morb Mortal Wkly Rep 2015;64(RR-3). Available at: https://www.cdc.gov/std/tg2015/syphilis.htm.
29. Hicks CB, Clement M. Syphilis: Treatment and monitoring. 2018. Up to Date website Available at: https://www.uptodate.com/contents/syphilis-treatment-and-monitoring?topicRef=7600&source=see_link. Accessed October 24, 2019.
30. U.S. Department of Health and Human Services. Poverty guidelines 2019. Available at: https://aspe.hhs.gov/2019-poverty-guidelines.
31. Healthy People 2020. Washington, DC: U.S. Department of Health and Human Services, Office of Disease Prevention and Health Promotion. Available at: https://www.healthypeople.gov/2020/topics-objectives/topic/sexually-transmitted-diseases. Accessed September 30,2019.

32. U.S. Department of Health and Human Services. Title X Planning. Office of Population Affairs. 2019. Available at: https://www.hhs.gov/opa/title-x-family-planning/index.html. Accessed October 23, 2019.
33. Frederiksen B, Salganicoff A, Gomez I, et al. Data not: impact of new Title X regulations on network participation. Kaiser Family Foundation. Available at: https://www.kff.org/womens-health-policy/issue-brief/data-note-impact-of-new-title-x-regulations-on-network-participation/. Accessed October 24, 2019.
34. Zule WA, Costenbader EC, Meyer WJ Jr, et al. Methamphetamine use and risky sexual behaviors during heterosexual encounters. Sex Transm Dis 2007;34:689–94.
35. Kidd SE, Grey JA, Torrone EA, et al. Increase methamphetamine, injection drug, and heroin use among women and heterosexual men with primary and secondary syphilis-United States, 2013-2017. MMWR Morb Mortal Wkly Rep 2018;68(6):144–8.
36. Yu J, Appel P, Rogers M, et al. Integrating intervention for substance use disorder in a healthcare setting: practice and outcomes in New York City STD clinics. Am J Drug Alcohol Abuse 2016;42:32–8.
37. Belluz J. Tinder and Grindr don't want to talk about their role in rising STDs. Vox Magazine 2017. Available at: https://www.vox.com/science-and-health/2017/11/13/16620286/online-dating-stds-tinder-grindr. Accessed November 12, 2019.
38. Tay L. Just 24 States Mandate Sex Education for K-12 Students, and Only 9 Require Any Discussion of Consent. See How Your State Stacks Up. 2019. Available at: https://www.the74million.org/article/just-24-states-mandate-sex-education-for-k-12-students-and-only-9-require-any-discussion-of-consent-see-how-your-state-stacks-up/.
39. de Voux A, Kidd S, Grey JA, et al. State-specific rates of primary and secondary syphilis among men who have sex with men—United States, 2015. MMWR Morb Mortal Wkly Rep 2017;66:349–54.
40. Mayer K. Old pathogen, new challenges: a narrative review of the multi-level drivers of syphilis increasing in American men who have sex with men. Sex Transm Dis 2018;45(9):s38–41.
41. Nath R, Grennan T, Parry R. Knowledge and attitudes of syphilis and syphilis pre-exposure prophylaxis (PrEP) among men who have sex with men in Vancouver, Canada: a qualitative study. BMJ Open 2019;9:e031239.
42. Kojima N, Dvora DJ, Klausner JD. Pre-exposure prophylaxis for HIV infection and new sexually transmitted infections among men who have sex with men. AIDS 2016;30(14):2251–2.
43. Traeger MW, Schroeder SE, Wright EJ, et al. Effects of pre-exposure prophylaxis for the prevention of human immunodeficiency virus infection on sexual risk behavior in men who have sex with men: A systematic review and meta-analysis. Clin Infect Dis 2018;67(5):676–86.
44. McCormack S, Dunn DT, Desai M, et al. Preexposure prophylaxis to prevent the acquisition of HIV-1 infection (PROUD): effectiveness results from the pilot phase of a pragmatic open-label randomised trial. Lancet 2016;387:53–60.
45. García-Legaz Martínez M, Hernández-Bel P, Magdaleno-Tapial J, et al. Usefulness of new automated treponemal tests in the diagnosis of early syphilis: a series of 15 cases. Actas Dermosifiliogr 2019;111(2):135–42.

The Use of Technology in the Management of Sexually Transmitted Infections

Angelina Anthamatten, DNP, FNP-BC*, Nicole Dellise, DNP, FNP-BC

KEYWORDS

• Sexually transmitted infection • Medical technology • Mobile application • App
• Medical reference • Point of care

KEY POINTS

- Several evidence-based resources may be accessed with technology to assist clinicians in screening, diagnosis, and management of sexually transmitted infections.
- Mobile medical technology can enhance health care professionals' access to updated, evidence-based clinical information in the office and at the point of care.
- Health care professionals should appraise the quality of medical information on the Internet and mobile medical applications and use clinical judgment when interpreting and applying the information.

BACKGROUND

There is a vast amount of evidence-based literature to inform clinical decision making. As technology has evolved, some of this evidence-based content has been integrated into Web sites and mobile applications ("apps") for smartphones and tablets to enhance access and efficiency for clinicians in the office and at the point of care. The World Health Organization defined mHealth (mobile health) as "medical and public health practice supported by mobile devices, such as mobile phones, patient monitoring devices, personal digital assistants (PDAs), and other wireless devices."[1(p6)] In a 2013 survey of more than 300 physicians practicing in primary care, family medicine, and internal medicine, 8 in 10 of these physicians reported using smartphones in their daily practice and 6 in 10 used tablets.[2] The top use of mobile technology for these respondents was accessing drug information (with smartphones) and accessing medical research (with tablets).[2] Many of these respondents used mobile devices to access to evidence-based clinical reference tools at the point of care with patients, with 50% using tablets and 42% using smartphones.[2] Another survey of

Vanderbilt University School of Nursing, 461 21st Avenue South, Nashville, TN 37240, USA
* Corresponding author:
E-mail address: angel.anthamatten@vanderbilt.edu

Nurs Clin N Am 55 (2020) 379–391
https://doi.org/10.1016/j.cnur.2020.06.002
0029-6465/20/© 2020 Elsevier Inc. All rights reserved.

approximately 3000 physicians revealed physicians' usage of smartphones for professional purposes in the United States increased from 68% in 2012 to 84% in 2015.[3] Wolters Kluwer health performed a survey for nurses in 2014 that explored the mobile device, Internet, and social media usage habits of nurse practitioners.[4] Sixty-five percent of these nurses reported currently using a mobile device for professional purposes at work.[4]

Mobile devices and applications are used by health care professionals in a variety of ways, including for reference and clinical decision making. These resources encompass medical literature, drug reference guides, clinical decision support systems, clinical treatment guidelines, disease diagnosis aids, medical calculators, and laboratory test interpretation.[5] Mobile devices can be of benefit if they allow more efficient access to evidence-based clinical information that has been vetted and is consistently updated.[4] Although many provide access to secure, trusted content, it is important that health care professionals remain cognizant that all Web sites and apps are not equivalent in quality.[4] Thus, a health care professional should appraise medical technology before use.

Some challenges related to using mobile medical resources are knowing what is available, where it is located, and the quality of the information. The purpose of this review was to provide an overview of some Web sites and mobile medical applications that can be used by health care providers for the management of a variety of sexually transmitted infections (STIs), such as trichomoniasis, chlamydia, gonorrhea, syphilis, genital herpes, human immunodeficiency virus (HIV), and hepatitis (**Table 1**). An overview of some practical strategies that health care professionals can use as they analyze the quality of information found on the Internet and mobile medical applications is also included (**Table 2**).

ACCESSING MEDICAL RESOURCES FOR MANAGEMENT OF SEXUALLY TRANSMITTED INFECTIONS WITH TECHNOLOGY
Sexually Transmitted Disease Treatment Guide Mobile Application

The STD (sexually transmitted disease) Tx (treatment) Guide by the Centers for Disease Control and Prevention (CDC) is a free mobile application for Apple iOS and Android devices that can serve as a quick reference guide for clinicians regarding identification and treatment of a variety of STIs.[6] The CDC's Division of STD Prevention and the Informatics Innovation Unit within CDC's Division of Public Health Information Dissemination–Center for Surveillance, Epidemiology and Laboratory Services collaborated in the development of this app.[6] There is a variety of information within this app, including 22 conditions, related terms and abbreviations, a guide to taking a sexual history, and a link to the CDC's treatment guidelines from 2015.[6] Specific treatment information is outlined and many topics have a tab for more information.[6] Pediatric and pregnancy considerations are also included for several topics.[6] According to the app for Apple iOS users, several updated versions have been published since 2015, with the most recent being in 2018 at the time of writing.[6] Updates regarding syphilis and drug-resistant gonorrhea are available at the CDC Web site.[7] The CDC Web site also has a wealth of patient education resources that clinicians can share.[8]

Sanford Guide to Antimicrobial Therapy Mobile Application

The Sanford Guide to Antimicrobial Therapy mobile application is a fee-based clinical reference for Apple iOS and Android devices that presents antimicrobial treatment options for a variety infectious processes, and it includes a section covering 10 STIs.[9]

Table 1
Examples of medical references that may be used with the management of sexually transmitted infections

Resource	Free or Cost	Content Overview	Access Information
CDC's STD Tx Guide	Free	Quick reference guide for health care professionals regarding the identification of and treatment for a variety of STIs	Mobile application for smartphone and tablet; Web site (https://www.cdc.gov/std/tg2015/default.htm)
Sanford Guide to Antimicrobial Therapy	Cost	Antimicrobial treatment recommendations for infectious conditions, including STIs	Mobile application for smartphone and tablet (https://www.sanfordguide.com/products/digital-subscriptions/sanford-guide-to-antimicrobial-therapy-mobile/); Web Edition (https://www.sanfordguide.com/products/digital-subscriptions/web-edition/)
Epocrates	Free (limited vers on); Cost (Epocrates plus full version)	Drug and prescribing information; drug interaction checker; pill identification; expanded content in full version, such as additional disease information and treatment guidance	Mobile application for smartphone and tablet (https://www.epocrates.com/products/features); Web site (https://online.epocrates.com)
Sanford Guide to HIV/AIDS Therapy	Cost	Information regarding the diagnosis and management of HIV/AIDS and related syndromes	Mobile application for smartphone and tablet (https://www.sanfordguide.com/products/digital-subscriptions/sanford-guide-to-hivaids-therapy-mobile/); Web Edition (https://www.sanfordguide.com/products/digital-subscriptions/web-edition/)
University of Liverpool's Resources for HIV	Free	Prescribing resources for HIV and drug interaction checker	Mobile application for smartphones and tablet; Web site (https://www.hiv-druginteractions.org/prescribing-resources; https://www.hiv-druginteractions.org/checker)

(continued on next page)

Table 1
(continued)

Resource	Free or Cost	Content Overview	Access Information
Johns Hopkins HIV guide	Cost	Information regarding the diagnosis and management of HIV	Web and mobile resource (https://www.unboundmedicine.com/products/johns_hopkins_hiv_guide)
HIV InSite (Center for HIV Information at the University of California San Francisco)	Free	HIV knowledge base, treatment information, drug interactions database	Website (http://hivinsite.ucsf.edu/InSite?page=ar-00-02)
HIV/HCV drug therapy guide (University Health Network)	Free	Drug and interaction information related to HIV and Hepatitis C therapies	Mobile application for smartphone and tablet; Web site (https://hivclinic.ca/wp-content/plugins/php/app.php)
Sanford Guide to Hepatitis Therapy	Cost	Information for the treatment of hepatitis A, B, and C	Mobile application for smartphone and tablet (https://www.sanfordguide.com/products/digital-subscriptions/sanford-guide-to-hepatitis-therapy-mobile/); Web Edition (https://www.sanfordguide.com/products/digital-subscriptions/web-edition/)
University of Liverpool's Resources for Hepatitis	Free	Prescribing resources for hepatitis and drug interaction checker	Mobile application for smartphone and tablet; Web site (https://www.hep-druginteractions.org/prescribing-resources)
GoodRx and GoodRx Pro	Free	Prescription discount resource; drug prices, coupons, alerts for refill reminders, drug information, pill images, pill identifier	Mobile application for smartphone and tablet; Web sites (https://www.goodrx.com; https://www.goodrx.com/professionals)

Abbreviations: CDC, Centers for Disease Control and Prevention; HCV, hepatitis C virus; HIV, human immunodeficiency virus; STD, sexually transmitted disease; STI, sexually transmitted infection.

Data from Refs.[6,9,11,19,21,23,25–27,29–32,34–38]

Table 2
Resources for evaluating medical information on the Internet and mobile medical applications

Resource	Target	Evaluation Criteria	Web Site Link
"HONcode: The commitment to reliable health and medical information on the Internet" (The Health on the New Foundation [HON])	Web sites	HON principles: authority, complementarity, confidentiality, attribution, justifiability, transparency, financial disclosure, and advertising	https://www.hon.ch/HONcode/Pro/Visitor/visitor.html
"Assessing the Quality of Internet Health Information" (The Agency for Healthcare Research and Quality [AHRQ])	Web sites	Credibility, content, disclosure, links, design, interactivity, caveats	https://archive.ahrq.gov/research/data/infoqual.html
"Evaluating Health Websites" (National Library of Medicine)	Web sites	Accuracy, authority, bias/objectivity, currency/timeliness, coverage	https://nnlm.gov/initiatives/topics/health-websites
"Evaluating Mobile Medical Applications" (Hanrahan et al,[42] 2014)	Mobile medical applications	Evaluation Tools: 1. Rubric for evaluating mobile drug information applications 2. Checklist for evaluating mobile drug information and medical reference applications 3. Checklist for evaluating mobile medical calculators	https://www.ashp.org/-/media/store%20files/mobile-medical-apps.pdf

Data from Refs.[39–42]

This app was developed by Antimicrobial Therapy, Inc. and offers primary and alternative regimens for many infectious processes, key points related to the disease and antimicrobial stewardship, as well as links to guidelines and references.[9] Many updated versions are noted within the app, with the most recent being late 2019 at the time of writing.[9] The Sanford Guide organization states they strive to improve patient care by providing clinicians with information that is accessible, concise, and reliable, and their editorial board consists of infectious disease experts from leading academic and clinical centers around the United States.[10]

Epocrates

There are several useful resources included within the Epocrates medical reference that may be helpful when treating an STI. Epocrates offers both a Web site and a mobile application for Apple iOS and Android devices, with free and fee-based versions that provide drug and disease clinical support.[11] Many updated versions of the app were noted at the time of writing, with the most recent being late 2019.[11] In the free version of this reference, professionals can find drug information, dosing recommendations, black box warnings, contraindications, cautions, common and significant adverse effects, a drug interaction checking tool, considerations for prescribing for pregnant or lactating women, pill identification, calculators, content from guidelines, and a variety of clinical reference tables.[11] There are expanded resources in the full version of Epocrates that may be purchased, such as additional disease content, access to antimicrobial treatment guidance, and laboratory information.[11] Because young people ages 15 to 24 years represent 50% of all new STIs,[12] clinicians may find Epocrates helpful for reviewing pediatric prescribing and dosing information.[11]

Medical Resources for Human Immunodeficiency Virus and Hepatitis

HIV and Hepatitis B virus (HBV) are bloodborne viruses that may be transmitted through sexual contact.[13] People who have an STI may be at an increased risk of getting HIV for a variety of reasons, and STIs can also increase the risk of spreading HIV.[14] Individuals with STIs are at least 2 to 5 times more likely to become infected with HIV when exposed through sexual contact.[15] In addition, a person living with HIV (PLWH) who is also infected with another STI is more likely than other PLWHs to transmit HIV through sexual contact.[15] Some STIs that are closely linked with HIV are syphilis, gonorrhea, and herpes simplex virus 2.[14] Appropriate treatment for HIV is essential, and health care professionals should be aware that there are frequent updates to recommendations found in the literature due to the dynamic nature of research.

Mobile applications have also been developed to assist clinicians caring for comorbid conditions in people living with HIV. Approximately 37 million individuals worldwide are living with HIV.[16] Although advances in therapy have yielded effective regimens, antiretroviral drugs have been described as being among the most therapeutically risky for drug-drug interactions (DDI).[16] DDIs can present significant risks to patients, thus they must be considered by health care providers to ensure safe and appropriate prescribing.[16] With new and improved antiretroviral therapies (ARTs), PLWHs are living longer and more primary care providers are involved in the management of comorbid chronic diseases and other routine primary care issues.[17,18] Because PLWHs are at particularly high risk of polypharmacy and DDIs, clinicians should be prepared to check for interactions and consider how the results affect clinical decisions.[17] It is important to use resources that provide continually updated prescribing information, due to the complexity of DDIs and the evolving nature of pharmacologic therapies and body of evidence.

Sanford guide to Human Immunodeficiency Virus/Acquired Immune Deficiency Syndrome therapy mobile application

The Sanford Guide to HIV/AIDS therapy application was developed by Antimicrobial Therapy, Inc. for Apple iOS and Android devices and offers detailed information regarding the diagnosis and management of HIV/AIDS and related syndromes, with content updated monthly.[19] Some topics include risk assessment, recommended testing, evaluation, HIV postexposure management, preexposure prophylaxis, immunizations, antiretroviral treatment, DDIs, cost comparison, drugs in development, HIV-related syndromes, pregnancy, newborn, and children.[19]

University of Liverpool's prescribing resources for human immunodeficiency virus

The University of Liverpool offers free robust HIV prescribing resources through their Web site, including comprehensive drug-drug interaction charts that are available on-line.[20] The Liverpool Drug Interactions Web site was established in 1999 by members of the Department of Pharmacology at the University of Liverpool to provide a freely available drug-drug interaction resource.[16] Their mission is to "provide a clinically useful, reliable, comprehensive, up-to-date, evidence-based drug-drug interaction resource, freely available to health care workers, patients, and researchers."[16(p1)]

The DDI charts in the University of Liverpool's prescribing resources are well-organized and include a vast amount of information.[21] The charts are organized by therapeutic indication (such as lipid-lowering), as well as by various HIV drug classes. These charts use a color-coded system to describe ascending levels of risk, which can be categorized as lowest (green), lower (yellow), moderate (orange), and high-risk (red).[22] Coadministration of drugs should be avoided with interactions in the high-risk category that is notated as red on the University of Liverpool's DDI charts.[22] For moderate-risk interactions, the risk may be mitigated with provider knowledge and action, such as close monitoring or alteration of drug dosage or timing of administration (Liverpool charts-drug and condition).[22] With the lower-risk option, the potential interaction is predicted to be of weak intensity and additional action, monitoring, or dosage adjustment is unlikely to be required (Liverpool charts-drug and condition).[22] For the lowest-risk category, no clinically significant interaction is expected (Liverpool chart).[22] Clinicians can also input specific drugs into their online drug interaction checker.[23]

This organization also offers drug information via mobile applications for Apple iOS and Android devices.[20] The University of Liverpool's Liverpool Drug Interactions Group and Clubzap Ltd. developed a free downloadable app that can be used in the office and at the point of care, with the most recent versions being from August 2018 at the time of writing.[24] It provides evidence-based information regarding potential drug-drug interactions between ART and other medications.[24] The mobile app offers an additional benefit of quality of evidence related to DDI results.[24] International treatment guidelines are used and a grading of the quality of evidence (very low, low, moderate, high) is reported for consideration by the health care professional.[24] Traffic light colors of red, amber, yellow, and green are used to present results and recommendations.[24]

Johns Hopkins human immunodeficiency virus guide

Unbound Medicine, Inc. collaborated with experts at Johns Hopkins Medicine to develop an HIV Web and mobile guide for Apple iOS and Android devices that is updated monthly and offers information regarding diagnosis, opportunistic infections, management options, clinical recommendations, adverse drug reactions, complications of treatment, and interactions.[25] Reference links for medical literature are also included within this resource.[25]

Human immunodeficiency virus InSite

Another Web site for HIV/AIDS and DDI information is HIV InSite, which was developed by the Center for HIV information at the University of California San Francisco. The organization states the site is edited by a physician and faculty member in the Division of HIV, ID & Global Medicine, updated daily, and offers comprehensive, up-to-date information on HIV/AIDS treatment and prevention.[26] The copyright is 2019 at the time of writing, but some various dates for content update were noted within the site.[26] Some of the content included in this Web site includes a knowledge base, treatment information, and a database of antiretroviral drug interactions searchable by antiretroviral drug, interacting drug, or interacting drug class.[26,27]

Human immunodeficiency virus/hepatitis C virus drug therapy guide

People living with HIV infection are disproportionally affected by viral hepatitis.[28] According to the CDC, approximately 25% of people with HIV in the United States are coinfected with hepatitis C virus (HCV) and approximately 10% are coinfected with HBV.[28] Hepatitis therapy is also dynamic, and clinicians must consider frequent updates. For individuals with HIV and HCV, the University Health Network–Toronto General Hospital, Immunodeficiency Clinic and collaborators developed a drug therapy guide that is available online and via free mobile applications for Apple iOS and Android devices.[29] The Web site was last updated in late 2019 at the time of writing, and the most recent version of the app was in 2017. This reference includes HIV and HCV drug information, as well as drug interaction tables that can be used when prescribing medications for common comorbid conditions, such as diabetes, dyslipidemia, hypertension, and depression.[30]

Sanford guide to hepatitis therapy mobile application

The Sanford guide also offers a mobile application for treatment of hepatitis A, B, and C that may be purchased with a subscription. The Sanford Guide to Hepatitis Therapy apps for Apple iOS and Android devices were developed by Antimicrobial Therapy, Inc. and designed to help clinicians stay abreast of current guidelines and options.[31] This reference provides comprehensive, regularly updated information on the prevention, management, and treatment of viral hepatitis infections.[31] Professionals can tap to access information that is organized by topic, or it can be queried using the full-text search function.[31]

University of Liverpool's prescribing resources for hepatitis

The University of Liverpool also offers a Web site and mobile application with prescribing resources for hepatitis.[32] The organization notes that "drug-drug interactions (DDIs) have the potential to cause harm due to liver dysfunction, multiple comorbidities, and comedications. This Web site was established in 2010 by members of the Department of Pharmacology at the University of Liverpool to offer a resource for health care providers, researchers and patients to be able to understand and manage drug-drug interactions...We actively promote the use of our Apps to health care providers and patients to enable rapid screening of DDIs."[33(p1)] Drug interaction charts provide an overview of interactions between direct-acting antivirals for HCV and the comedications listed in the interaction checker and color-coded clinical recommendations.[34]

GoodRx PRESCRIPTION DISCOUNT RESOURCE

Cost is an important factor in prescribing and can have a significant influence on medication adherence. The GoodRx Web site and mobile applications for Apple iOS and

Android devices are free and provide current prices and discounts to help patients and health care professionals find the lowest-cost pharmacy for prescription drugs.[35,36] A patient may also find a GoodRx coupon to redeem at the pharmacy of their choice and reduce the cash price of a prescription.[35] Two versions of the mobile application have been developed by GoodRx: GoodRx for patients, with a most recent version in late 2019 at the time of writing, and GoodRx Pro for health care professionals, updated in 2018.[37,38] In addition to drug cost and discount information, the patient version offers a pill identifier and alerts for refill reminders and lower prices.[37] Patients and health care professionals can also find pill images, information on recalls by the Food and Drug Administration (FDA), and drug information from Truven Health Micromedex that is included as an educational aid, such as how to administer the drug, what to do if a dose is missed, storage recommendations, what to watch for, potential adverse effects, and interaction considerations.[35,37,38]

Appraising the Quality of Medical Information on the Internet and Mobile Applications

Mobile medical resources can be a helpful and efficient aid for clinicians. However, it is essential that clinicians appraise the credibility of the developer and quality of information. There are frequent developments in research and updates in evidence-based recommendations.

Thus, clinicians should also determine how these updates are incorporated into each mobile resource. Many medical applications and Web sites also include a variety of disclaimers, such as limitations of information presented, need for clinicians to confirm information and exercise their own judgment when interpreting and applying the information, and other legal considerations. Privacy policies, license agreements, and support can also be found within mobile applications.

Several tools are available to appraise the quality and accuracy of electronic medical resources. **Table 2** outlines several resources that can be used to assist medical professionals in systematic evaluation of medical information on the Internet and mobile medical applications. The Health on the New Foundation (HON) is one example.[39] HON is a nongovernmental organization, internationally known for its pioneering work in the field of health information ethics, notably for the establishment of its code of ethical conduct, the HONcode.[39] The HON Code of Conduct uses the following 8 criteria to evaluate medical and health Web sites: authority, complementarity, confidentiality, attribution, justifiability, transparency, financial disclosure, and advertising.[39] Web sites may request a "HONcode seal" to be placed on the site, and, if awarded, HON conducts regular monitoring to ensure compliance with the 8 principles.[39] The Agency for Healthcare Research and Quality and the National Library of Medicine also developed evaluation criteria to provide guidance in determining Web site quality.[40,41] Although helpful, these resources do not specifically target mobile applications at this time. Due to rapid technology growth and mobile application advancement, tools to assess the quality of mobile applications are limited. Using several concepts from tools used to assess electronic medical resources, Hanrahan and colleagues[42] developed comprehensive checklists and evaluation rubrics that may be applied to appraisal of mobile applications. The FDA has also published guidance to provide clarity on the scope of their oversight of clinical decision support software intended for health care professionals, patients, or caregivers.[43] The guidance is intended to inform app developers about regulation related to clinical decision support apps that provide diagnostic and treatment recommendations to health care professionals.[43,44] Clinical decision support apps are distinct and differ from patient decision support apps, which provide information only to the patient.[44]

The focus of this review was medical resources for health care professionals. However, just as health care professionals should appraise quality of mobile medical technology before use, professionals also have a responsibility to critically evaluate mHealth apps they may recommend to their patients.[45] A simple checklist tool was developed for physicians to assess quality of mobile health applications before discussing their use with patients.[45]

SUMMARY

Several evidence-based resources may be accessed with technology to assist clinicians in screening, diagnosis, and management of sexually transmitted infections. Medical information on the Internet and mobile medical applications can provide helpful and efficient resources for clinicians. However, it is essential that clinicians appraise the quality of this technology and use clinical judgment when interpreting and applying the information. This review includes an overview of several clinical resources for health care professionals, but these are only examples of what is available. According to a mHealth app developer economics study, 325,000 mobile health applications were available in 2017.[46] Because this is a significant and developing area of interest for health care professionals and the public, professionals will likely find many opportunities to use the strategies presented to identify resources and evaluate the quality of health and medical technology they would like to use in their clinical practices.

DISCLOSURE

The authors have nothing to disclose.

REFERENCES

1. World Health Organization. mHealth: New horizons for health through mobile technologies. Available at: https://www.who.int/goe/publications/goe_mhealth_web.pdf. Accessed December 21, 2019.
2. Wolters Kluwer Health. Wolters Kluwer Health 2013 physician outlook survey. Available at: http://wolterskluwer.com/binaries/content/assets/wk-health/pdf/company/newsroom/white-papers/wolters-kluwer-health-physician-study-executive-summary.pdf. Accessed December 20, 2019.
3. Statista Research Department. Smartphone use for professional reasons among U.S. physicians 2012-2015. 2016. Available at: https://www.statista.com/statistics/416951/smartphone-use-for-professional-purposes-among-us-physicians/. Accessed December 20, 2019.
4. Wolters Kluwer Health. Wolters Kluwer Health survey finds nurses and healthcare institutions accepting professional use of online reference & mobile technology. 2014. Available at: https://wolterskluwer.com/company/newsroom/news/health/2014/09/wolters-kluwer-health-survey-finds-nurses-and-healthcare-institutions-accepting-professional-use-of-online-reference–mobile-technology.html. Accessed December 20, 2019.
5. Ventola CL. Mobile devices and apps for health care professionals: uses and benefits. P T 2014;39(5):356–64.
6. Centers for Disease Control and Prevention. CDC STD Tx Guide. Version 2.4.1.6 [Apple iOS application]. Accessed July 5, 2019. 2019.
7. U.S. Department of Health & Human Services. Sexually transmitted diseases-treatment and screening. Centers for Disease Control and Prevention; 2013. Available at: https://www.cdc.gov/std/treatment/. Accessed December 2, 2019.

8. U.S. Department of Health & Human Services. Sexually transmitted diseases-CDC fact sheets. Centers for Disease Control and Prevention Website; 2016. Available at: https://www.cdc.gov/std/healthcomm/fact_sheets.htm. Accessed December 2, 2019.
9. Antimicrobial Therapy Inc. Sanford guide to antimicrobial therapy. Version 4.0.3. [Apple iOS application]. Accessed July 5, 2019.
10. Sanford Guide. About us. Available at: https://www.sanfordguide.com/about/. Accessed December 20, 2019.
11. Epocrates. Version 19.12. [Apple iOS application]. Accessed July 5, 2019.
12. U.S. Department of Health & Human Services. Sexually transmitted diseases-STD prevention infographics. Centers for Disease Control and Prevention; 2015. Available at: https://www.cdc.gov/std/products/infographics.htm#EPTinfographic. Accessed December 2, 2019.
13. U.S. Department of Health & Human Services. Viral hepatitis. Centers for Disease Control and Prevention; 2019. Available at: https://www.cdc.gov/hepatitis/populations/hiv.htm. Accessed December 2, 2019.
14. U.S. Department of Health & Human Services. HIV/AIDS and STDs. Centers for Disease Control and Prevention; 2019. Available at: https://www.cdc.gov/std/hiv/stdfact-std-hiv-detailed.htm. Accessed December 2, 2019.
15. U.S. Department of Health & Human Services. The role of STD prevention and treatment in HIV prevention. Centers for Disease Control and Prevention; 2010. Available at: https://www.cdc.gov/std/hiv/stds-and-hiv-fact-sheet.pdf. Accessed February 19, 2020.
16. University of Liverpool. Mission statement. 2019. Available at: https://www.hivdruginteractions.org/mission. Accessed July 5, 2019-December 21, 2019.
17. Hughes CA, Tseng A, Cooper R. Managing drug interactions in HIV-infected adults with comorbid illness. Can Med Assoc J 2015;187(1):36–43.
18. Non LR, Escota GV, Powderly WG. HIV and its relationship to insulin resistance and lipid abnormalities. Transl Res 2017;183:41–56.
19. Sanford Guide. HIV/AIDS therapy app. Available at: https://www.sanfordguide.com/products/digital-subscriptions/sanford-guide-to-hivaids-therapy-mobile/?_ga=2.264585352.64034102.1576882317-1664032774.1576880561. Accessed December 20, 2019.
20. University of Liverpool. HIV drug interactions. 2019. Available at: https://www.hiv-druginteractions.org/. Accessed May 20, 2019–December 21, 2019.
21. University of Liverpool. HIV drug interactions-prescribing resources. 2019. Available at: https://www.hiv-druginteractions.org/prescribing-resources. Accessed May 20, 2019–December 21, 2019.
22. University of Liverpool. HIV drug interactions-lipid-lowering treatment selector. 2019. Available at: https://liverpool-hiv-hep.s3.amazonaws.com/prescribing_resources/pdfs/000/000/031/original/TS_LipidLowering_2019_Dec.pdf?1575369382. Accessed December 20, 2019.
23. University of Liverpool. HIV drug interactions. 2019. Available at: https://www.hiv-druginteractions.org/checker. Accessed May 20, 2019–December 21, 2019.
24. Liverpool drug interactions group. Liverpool HIV iChart. 2018. Available at: https://apps.apple.com/gb/app/liverpool-hiv-ichart/id979962744; https://play.google.com/store/apps/details?id=com.liverpooluni.icharthiv&hl=en_GB. Accessed July 5, 2019.
25. Unbound Medicine. Johns Hopkins HIV guide. Available at: https://www.unboundmedicine.com/products/johns_hopkins_hiv_guide. Accessed December 20, 2019.

26. Center for HIV Information- University of California, San Francisco. HIV InSite. Available at: https://hividgm.ucsf.edu/hiv-insite http://hivinsite.ucsf.edu/InSite. Accessed December 21, 2019.

27. Center for HIV Information- University of California, San Francisco. Database of antiretroviral drug interactions. Available at: http://hivinsite.ucsf.edu/InSite?page=ar-00-02. Accessed December 20, 2019.

28. U.S. Department of Health & Human Services. HIV and viral hepatitis. Centers for Disease Control and Prevention; 2017. Available at: https://www.cdc.gov/hiv/pdf/library/factsheets/hiv-viral-hepatitis.pdf. Accessed December 2, 2019.

29. University Health Network–Toronto General Hospital, Immunodeficiency Clinic. HIV/HCV Drug Therapy Guide. 2019. Available at: http://app.hivclinic.ca/. Accessed July 5, 2019–December 21, 2019.

30. University Health Network–Toronto General Hospital, Immunodeficiency Clinic. Drug Interaction Tables. Available at: https://hivclinic.ca/drug-information/drug-interaction-tables/. Accessed December 20, 2019.

31. Sanford Guide. Hepatitis Therapy App. Available at: https://www.sanfordguide.com/products/digital-subscriptions/sanford-guide-to-hepatitis-therapy-mobile/. Accessed July 5, 2019.

32. University of Liverpool. HEP drug interactions-prescribing resources. 2019. Available at: https://www.hep-druginteractions.org/prescribing-resources. Accessed July 5, 2019–December 21, 2019.

33. University of Liverpool. HEP drug interactions-mission statement. Available at: https://www.hep-druginteractions.org/mission. Accessed July 5, 2019.

34. University of Liverpool. HEP Drug Interactions-Interpreting the Liverpool HEP Interactions checker. Available at: https://liverpool-hiv-hep.s3.amazonaws.com/prescribing_resources/pdfs/000/000/134/original/ASHM_Interpreting_Liverpool_HEP_FINAL.pdf?1576835949. Accessed December 20, 2019.

35. GoodRx. Available at: https://www.goodrx.com https://www.goodrx.com/professionals. Accessed December 20, 2019.

36. GoodRx. Good Rx mobile apps. Available at: https://www.goodrx.com/mobile. Accessed December 20, 2019.

37. GoodRx. Version 5.4.3. [Apple iOS application]. Accessed November 4, 2019. 2019.

38. GoodRx Pro. Version 1.5 [Apple iOS application]. Accessed November 4, 2019. 2019.

39. Health on the Net. HON code. 2017. Available at: https://www.hon.ch/HONcode/Pro/Visitor/visitor.html. Accessed December 1, 2019.

40. U. S. Department of Health & Human Services. Assessing the quality of Internet health information. Agency for Healthcare Research and Quality. 1999. Available at: https://archive.ahrq.gov/research/data/infoqual.html. Accessed December 1, 2019.

41. U.S. Department of Health & Human Services. Evaluating health websites. National Network of Libraries of Medicine. Available at: https://nnlm.gov/initiatives/topics/health-websites. Accessed December 1, 2019.

42. Hanrahan C, Augnst TD, Cole S. Evaluating mobile medical applications. Bethesda (MD): American Society of Health Systems Pharmacists; 2014. Available at: https://www.ashp.org/-/media/store%20files/mobile-medical-apps.pdf. Accessed December 1, 2019.

43. United States Food and Drug Administration. Clinical decision support software: guidance for industry and food and drug administration staff. 2019. Available at:

https://www.fda.gov/regulatory-information/search-fda-guidance-documents/clinical-decision-support-software. Accessed December 21, 2019.

44. Larson RS. A path to better-quality mHealth apps. J Med Internet Res 2018;6(7): e10414.
45. Cook VE, Ellis AK, Hildebrand KJ. Mobile health applications in clinical practice: pearls, pitfalls, and key considerations. Ann Allergy Asthma Immunol 2016; 117(2):143–9.
46. Research2Guidance. 325,000 mobile health apps available in 2017- android now the leading mHealth platform. Available at: https://research2guidance.com/325000-mobile-health-apps-available-in-2017/%202017. Accessed December 21, 2019.

Decreasing Barriers to Sexual Health in the Lesbian, Gay, Bisexual, Transgender, and Queer Community

Justin M. Waryold, DNP, RN, ANP-C, ACNP-BC, GS-C, CNE[a,b,*],
Allyson Kornahrens, DNP, RN, FNP-C, ENP-C, CNL, CRN, CCRN[c]

KEYWORDS

- Bisexual • Cultural awareness • Gay • Lesbian • Provider bias • Queer
- Sexual health • Transgender

KEY POINTS

- Providers need to show cultural competency in the care of lesbian, gay, bisexual, transgender, and queer individuals in an attempt to eradicate barriers to care for this population.
- Introducing environmental modifications assists in promoting an inclusive atmosphere.
- Alterations to the intake process and medical intake forms will support the patient's sense of belonging.
- When using a systematic approach for obtaining a sexual health history, providers can attain relevant clinical information in a culturally competent manner.

DECREASING BARRIERS TO SEXUAL HEALTH IN THE LESBIAN, GAY, BISEXUAL, TRANSGENDER, AND QUEER COMMUNITY

Instituting efforts to increase access to and improve the delivery of culturally competent health care for sexual minorities has been noted as a priority of Healthy People 2020, the Institute of Medicine (IOM), and the Agency for Healthcare Research and Quality.[1–3] This concept applies to the lesbian, gay, bisexual, transgender, and queer

[a] Department of Graduate Studies: Adult Health, Stony Brook University School of Nursing, 101 Nichols Road, HSC Level 2, Room 222, Stony Brook, NY 11794, USA; [b] Department of Medicine, Stony Brook University School of Medicine, 101 Nichols Road, HSC Level 2, Room 222, Stony Brook, NY 11794, USA; [c] Department of Graduate Studies: Family Health, Stony Brook University School of Nursing, 101 Nichols Road, HSC Level 2, Room 213-C, Stony Brook, NY 11794, USA
* Corresponding author. Stony Brook University School of Nursing, HSC, Level 2, Room 222, Stony Brook, NY 11794-8240.
E-mail address: Justin.waryold@stonybrook.edu

Nurs Clin N Am 55 (2020) 393–402
https://doi.org/10.1016/j.cnur.2020.06.003
0029-6465/20/© 2020 Elsevier Inc. All rights reserved.
nursing.theclinics.com

(LGBTQ+) populations in particular. The symbol of plus (+) is added to the acronym to expand the reach to people of all gender identities and sexual orientations.[4] Recognition within the 2011 IOM report remarked that each letter represents a distinctive population accompanied by its own health disparities.[5,6] A barrier to quality health care for this community lies in locating a provider who not only is knowledgeable of concerns specific to those in the LGBTQ+ community but also provides care in an environment that is open and welcoming.

BACKGROUND

In recent years, increased acceptance of the LGBTQ+ community has fostered an opportunity for individuals to be open about their sexuality, allowing them to present as their authentic selves. In the 2017 Gallup Poll, approximately 4.5% of adult respondents who live in the United States identified as LGBTQ+, with an estimated total that may exceed 11 million people in the United States. This number is an increase from 3.5% in 2012.[7] The increase in the LGBTQ+ population dictates the necessity for culturally competent providers to address the specific health needs of these individuals.

The opportunity for members of the LGBTQ+ community to access knowledgeable practitioners within a safe and welcoming environment continues to be problematic. Finding culturally competent care is challenging for these individuals. Instances of outright discrimination, perceived inadequate or inappropriate care, and ineffective communication have been reported.[8–12] Transgender individuals, in particular, have reported experiences of discrimination within the health care arena because of their gender identity, whereas others anticipate discrimination, resulting in an avoidance of care.[11,13] These occurrences can contribute to a deterioration in health, because they potentially limit opportunities for care.[13] Regular, routine, and preventive care are of great importance because of the higher incidence of certain types of cancer and exacerbation of chronic illnesses experienced by the LGBTQ+ individuals.[5] Avoiding care is a contributing factor in delaying appropriate treatment and has resulted in substandard care for LGBTQ individuals.[10,14]

ADDRESSING PROVIDER BIAS

Biases can exist in the conscious or unconscious mind. Explicit biases are consciously controlled and tend to be susceptible to social influence, particularly when others share the same views on the matter.[15] This type of bias is expressed openly and occupies the conscious mind. Implicit biases are automatic responses that occur beyond conscious thinking and may contribute to inequitable care.[16] Providers may be unaware of these implicit biases, having no malicious intent regarding to whom they are directed.

Both implicit and explicit bias have the potential to affect communication between providers and their patients, potentially altering the providers' decision making. Providers can reduce the contribution of implicit bias by recognizing personal vulnerability and adopting skills such as individuation and perspective taking.[16] Use of strategies such as self-reflection, case scenario review, and collaboration with colleagues who provide care to LGBTQ+ individuals may better prepare providers. Although there is no existing training to eliminate implicit biases fully, stereotyping can be unlearned, and acknowledgment of these implicit biases can minimize their impact.[17] **Table 1**[4,15,17–20] provides a list of strategies for addressing and reducing implicit bias.

Table 1
Strategies in addressing and reducing implicit bias

Project Implicit: Implicit Association Test	The Implicit Association Test measures attitudes and beliefs that people may be unwilling or unable to report: https://implicit.harvard.edu/implicit/
Stereotype replacement	During your interaction with the individual, recognize that your response may be based on a stereotype and consciously adjusting the response
Individualization	Consciously seeing the person as an individual rather than a stereotypical group
Perspective taking	Allowing yourself to be "in their shoes"; how would you feel if you were placed in their situation?
Using case scenarios to address implicit biases	Developed by the National LGBT Health Education Center, this guide can help providers develop an awareness of their implicit biases via case scenarios: https://www.lgbthealtheducation.org/wp-content-uploads/2018/10/Implicit-Bias-Guide-2018_Final.pdf
Educate yourself about the specific health care needs of LGBTQ+ individuals	Examine self-paced educational modules to help you understand the underserved needs of this population: https://www.lgbthealtheducation.org/
Increase your exposure and opportunities to care for LGBTQ+ individuals	Seek out opportunities to network with colleagues who have an established practice caring for LGBTQ+ individuals

Data from Refs.[4,15,17–20]

CLINICAL ENVIRONMENT

The clinical setting should be a welcoming, safe environment for all persons who seek care at the practice. Subtle signs of inclusivity affirm, to patients, staff, and stakeholders alike, a practice that is friendly to the LGBTQ+ community. These signs may include a prominent display of the office's nondiscrimination policy and a rainbow flag at the intake window. Restrooms with "All Gender Restroom" signage provide access to all persons regardless of gender identity or expression. The display of rainbow flag pins or stickers on the identification badges of staff members and providers also signifies an inclusive environment and knowledgeable, welcoming staff.[21–25] **Table 2** summarizes suggested environmental adaptations. Although these interventions may seem trivial, the impact is vast and lasting for individuals who are seeking care.

PROVIDER MEDICAL FORMS AND INTAKE DOCUMENTS

Following environmental assessment and subsequent modifications, the practice must examine the health care documents and office logistics. Evaluation of the patient intake process is essential, beginning with the initial phone contact. Providers and practice staff should be aware that individuals may have preferred names that differ from their legal names, which may appear on medical records, legal documents,

Table 2
Suggestions for modifications of the clinical environment

Clinical Modification	Rational
Prominent display of organizational nondiscrimination policy	Alerts all individuals that the organization does not support or endorse discrimination. Equal care is provided to all persons, regardless of age, race, ethnicity, physical ability or attributes, region, sexual orientation, or gender identity/expression
LGBTQ+ friendly signage, such as rainbow stickers	Signifies an environment of care that welcomes the LGBTQ+ community
Gender-neutral restroom signage, "All gender restroom"	Promotes an inclusive environment, signifies that all individuals are welcomed and respected
Rainbow pins/stickers on staff identity badges	Signifies staff is educated to provide culturally competent care to members of the LGBTQ+ community
Display brochures (multilingual when possible) on health concerns relevant to the LGBTQ+ community, such as safe sex, breast cancer, hormone therapy, mental health, and sexually transmitted infections	Signifies a health community that is welcoming and inclusive
Display wall art depicting racially and ethnically diverse same-sex couples or transgender people	Promotes inclusivity within the environment
Acknowledge relevant days of observance in the practice, such as World AIDS Day, LGBT Pride Day, and National Transgender Day of Remembrance	Promotes awareness of LGBTQ+ history

government-issued identification, and insurance documents. Although electronic health record (EHR) systems vary, personnel need to be provided with education to enter an individual's preferred name into the appropriate fields.

The intake process also includes many informational forms to be completed by the patients or their representatives. These forms should use gender-neutral and inclusive language, providing adequate space for open-ended questions. These questions may relate to sexual orientation, gender identity, sex assigned at birth, as well as the preferred name. The availability of ample space for responses is a clear demonstration of an inclusive environment. In order to promote the inclusion of transgender or gender-nonconforming individuals, intake forms should include an organ inventory. This inventory provides a means to maintain a list of a patient's medical transition history and current anatomy[26], and can be updated as needed, alerting the provider on specific anatomy. **Box 1**[26] provides a list of organs for inventory to include on intake forms.

For intake processes that use the EHR, the availability of additional categories to promote inclusivity may not be as easily achieved. However, collaboration with the organizational EHR management may provide opportunities to improve the process. It is essential to note that this information is provided voluntarily, and further discussion can occur between the person and the provider. All staff should reiterate that this, as well as any information obtained, will be kept confidential.[5,27,28] **Box 2** includes suggested questions to be included in the EHR.

Box 1
Organs for inventory

- Penis
- Testicles
- Prostate
- Breasts
- Vagina
- Cervix
- Uterus
- Ovaries

From Deutsch MB, Green J, Keatley J, et al. Electronic medical records and the transgender patient: recommendations from the World Professional Association for Transgender Health EMR Working Group. *J Am Med Inform Assoc.* 2013;20(4):700-703; with permission.

VISIT WITH THE PROVIDER

On entrance into the examination room, individuals routinely experience increased apprehension and stress relating to the impending encounter. LGBTQ+ individuals may have increased trepidation because of perceived bias based on past experiences of poor communication and disrespectful behaviors during health care encounters.[8] The application of strategies to signify an inclusive environment before the examination room the patient encounters may reduce patient apprehension and foster an open dialogue between the patient and the provider. During the initial encounter, the provider should inquire about the patient's preferred name and pronouns, which may differ from those associated with the gender assigned at birth. These pronouns may be familiar (eg, his/hers) or may be gender neutral (them/their, zie/hir). The use of an individual's preferred name and pronouns signifies a respectful and affirming clinical environment, creating a foundation for a meaningful rapport between the

---

Box 2
Electronic health record sexual orientation and gender identity questions

Do you think yourself as:
- Lesbian, gay, or homosexual
- Straight or heterosexual
- Bisexual
- Do not know
- Not sure
- Choose not to disclose
- Other:

What is your current gender identity?
- Male
- Female
- Transgender man/transman
- Transgender woman/transwoman
- Genderqueer, neither exclusively male nor female
- Not sure
- Choose not to disclose
- Other:

patient and provider.[27,29] **Table 3**[30] provides a list of standard and gender-nonconforming pronouns.

The evaluation of the patient is similar to any other patient encounter. Individuals presenting for an assessment of a concern that may be of a sexual nature may be apprehensive about sharing their concerns in fear of discrimination, inappropriate or insensitive questioning, or unnecessary examination.[31] To help a provider formulate the appropriate questions and present them in a considerate matter, the PLISSIT (permission, limited information, specific suggestions, intensive therapy) model is a valuable tool. This model is an established method that assists providers in asking relevant questions in a respectful and nonjudgmental manner while offering consistency to ensure the acquisition of a thorough history.[32] **Table 4** provides a detailed overview of the PLISSIT model in the clinical setting. The initial query should include permission to ask questions about sexual health and concerns. It is essential to inform the patient that these questions are asked to all persons, regardless of sexual orientation, gender identification, or self-expression. This query is followed by obtaining limited information as it pertains to the concern. Allow the patients to speak freely and openly as they provide information that they think is relevant. The provider may guide the patient to help explore what is clinically relevant to the concern and limit the information needed for the evaluation.[33] Those identifying as transgender or gender nonconforming may not acknowledge anatomic parts or may use other terms for their anatomy. Providers can refer to the organ inventory to help frame clinically relevant questions. Inquiring in this format allows the provider to see people as their authentic selves and not categorize their sexual orientations or gender identifications. The provider provides specific suggestions in an understanding manner that address the concern. Lastly, intensive therapy allow the provider to consult appropriate referrals as needed.[33] Using the PLISSIT model helps providers obtain clinically relevant information in a matter that is respectful and continues to affirm each person's authentic self.

PROVIDER EDUCATION, RESOURCES, AND REFERRALS

As previously discussed, provider education may aid in increased cultural competency and increase provider preparedness for the care of LGBTQ+ individuals. Additional resources are summarized in **Table 5**.

In support of decreasing barriers to care, culturally competent providers that wish to promote their LGBTQ+ friendly practices are encouraged to consider enrolling in the Gay and Lesbian Medical Association's provider directory (https://glma.org/referrals).

Table 3				
Standard and unique pronouns				
He	Him	His	His	Himself
He studied	I called him	His pencil	That is his	He trusts himself
She	Her	Her	Hers	Herself
She studied	I called her	Her pencil	That is hers	She trusts herself
They	Them	Their	Theirs	Themselves
They studied	I called them	Their pencil	That is theirs	They trust themselves
Ze (or Zie)	Hir	Hir	Hirs	Hirself
Ze studied (zee)	I called hir (heer)	Hir pencil	That is hirs	Ze trusts hirself

Data from University of California San Francisco. Pronouns matter. Published 2019. Available at: https://lgbt.ucsf.edu/pronounsmatter. Accessed November 4, 2019.

Table 4
The PLISSIT model for interviewing

Abbreviation	Description	Explanation	Example
P	Permission	Obtain permission to discuss the sexual concern	"I would like to ask you some questions about your concern. These questions are of a personal nature about your sexual health. Your answers will help me better understand your concerns and help me provide better care to you. Would you mind answering these questions?"
LI	Limited information	Limit the inquiry about the sexual concern	"Can you describe what you are feeling? What activity did you engage in that makes you believe you are at risk for a sexually transmitted infection? When you are with your partner or partners, what body part touches what body part?"
SS	Specific suggestions	Provide specific suggestions to address the concern	"There are barriers that can be used during sex that can help protect you against sexually transmitted infections. In addition, there are vaccinations and medications can help reduce and even prevent some illnesses."
IT	Intensive therapy	Identify whether further expert consultation is required	"Some people find it helpful to explore these concerns further with a specialist. Would you be open to seeing someone who specializes in this area?"

Table 5
Provider resources

Resource	Web Site
The National LGBT Health Education Center	https://www.lgbthealtheducation.org/ Publications https://www.lgbthealtheducation.org/resources/type/ publication/ Learning modules https://www.lgbthealtheducation.org/resources/type/ learning-module/ Taking routine histories of sexual health: a system-wide approach for health centers https://www.lgbthealtheducation.org/wp-content/ uploads/COM-827-sexual-history_toolkit_2015.pdf
WPATH: World Professional Association for Transgender Health	https://www.wpath.org/ WPATH Standards of Care https://www.wpath.org/publications/soc
UCSF Transgender Care	https://transcare.ucsf.edu/ Guidelines for the Primary and Gender-Affirming Care of Transgender and Gender Nonbinary People https://transcare.ucsf.edu/guidelines
National Coalition for Sexual Health	https://nationalcoalitionforsexualhealth.org/ Sexual Health and Your Patients: A Provider's Guide https://nationalcoalitionforsexualhealth.org/tools/for-healthcare-providers/document/ProviderGuide.pdf
GLMA: Health Professionals Advancing LGBTQ Equality (previously known as the Gay and Lesbian Medical Association)	http://www.glma.org/ Guidelines for care of lesbian, gay, bisexual, and transgender patients https://www.rainbowwelcome.org/uploads/pdfs/GLMA% 20guidelines%202006%20FINAL.pdf
Parents, Family, and Friends of Lesbians and Gays	https://pflag.org/ Straight for Equality in Healthcare: https://www.straightforequality.org/Healthcare
National Organization of Nurse Practitioner Faculties: Patient-Centered Transgender Health	A Toolkit for Nurse Practitioner Faculty and Clinicians https://cdn.ymaws.com/www.nonpf.org/resource/resmgr/ files/transgender_toolkit_final.pdf
ACT for Youth Center for Community Action	http://actforyouth.net/ Resources for working with LGBT patients http://actforyouth.net/adolescence/healthcare/lgbt.cfm

This free, national directory encompasses a variety of providers, specialists, therapists, dentists, and other health professionals searched by location. This directory is equally vital to providers who provide care to LGBTQ+ individuals and have a patient who requires a consultation with a specialist (eg, psychological services). Using directories such as this, as well as having a referral network of LGBTQ+ friendly providers, will continue to decrease barriers to care and promote overall well-being.

SUMMARY

To provide adequate health care to the LGBTQ+ community, there must first be initiatives to diminish and eliminate health care disparities. Initial steps include the consideration of provider bias; the establishment of an inclusive environment; respectful communication using an individual's preferred name and preferred pronouns; and offering safe, meaningful, and appropriate screening that is individualized and free from assumption. The incorporation of these initiatives can aid in the elimination of barriers to care for all individuals who are seeking safe, appropriate, and individualized care.

DISCLOSURE

The authors have nothing to disclose.

REFERENCES

1. U.S. Department of Health and Human Services OoDPaHP. Healthy people 2020: lesbian, gay, bisexual, and transgender health 2019. Available at: https://www.healthypeople.gov/2020/topics-objectives/topic/lesbian-gay-bisexual-and-transgender-health. Accessed December 29, 2019.
2. Daniel H, Butkus R, Health ft. Physicians PPCotACo. Lesbian, Gay, bisexual, and transgender health disparities: executive summary of a policy position paper from the American College of Physicians. Ann Intern Med 2015;163(2):135–7.
3. Foglia MB, Fredriksen-Goldsen KI. Health disparities among LGBT older adults and the role of nonconscious bias. Hastings Cent Rep 2014;44:S40–4.
4. Wang-Jones TTS, Hauson AO, Ferdman BM, et al. Comparing implicit and explicit attitudes of gay, straight, and non-monosexual groups toward transmen and transwomen. Int J Transgend 2018;19(1):95–106.
5. Graham R, Berkowitz B, Blum R, et al. The health of lesbian, gay, bisexual, and transgender people: Building a foundation for better understanding. Washington, DC: Institute of Medicine; 2011.
6. The Human Rights Campaign. Glossary of terms. 2019. Available at: https://www.hrc.org/resources/glossary-of-terms. Accessed June 7, 2019.
7. Newport F. U.S., Estimate of LGBT Population Rises to 4.5%. Gallup. 2018. Available at: https://news.gallup.com/poll/234863/estimate-lgbt-population-rises.aspx. Accessed September 2, 2019.
8. Snyder BK, Burack GD, Petrova A. LGBTQ youth's perceptions of primary care. Clin Pediatr 2017;56(5):443–50.
9. Snyder M. Health care experiences of lesbian women: a metasynthesis. Adv Nurs Sci 2019;42(1):E1–22.
10. Rounds K, Burns Mcgrath B, Walsh E. Perspectives on provider behaviors: A qualitative study of sexual and gender minorities regarding quality of care. Contemp Nurse 2013;44(1):99–110.
11. Austin A, Craig SL. Transgender affirmative cognitive behavioral therapy: clinical considerations and applications. Prof Psychol Res Pract 2015;46(1):21–9.
12. Quinn GP, Sanchez JA, Sutton SK, et al. Cancer and lesbian, gay, bisexual, transgender/transsexual, and queer/questioning (LGBTQ) populations. CACancer J Clin 2015;65(5):384–400.
13. Casey LS, Reisner SL, Findling MG, et al. Discrimination in the United States: Experiences of lesbian, gay, bisexual, transgender, and queer Americans. Health Serv Res 2019;54:1454–66.
14. Sabin JA, Riskind RG, Nosek BA. Health care providers' implicit and explicit attitudes toward lesbian women and gay men. Am J Public Health 2015;105(9):1831–41.
15. Burke SE, Dovidio JF, Przedworski JM, et al. Do contact and empathy mitigate bias against gay and lesbian people among heterosexual first-year medical

students? a report from the medical student CHANGE study. Acad Med 2015; 90(5):645–51.

16. Chapman EN, Kaatz A, Carnes M. Physicians and implicit bias: how doctors may unwittingly perpetuate health care disparities. J Gen Intern Med 2013;28(11): 1504–10.

17. Wyatt R, Laderman M, Botwinick L, et al. Achieving health equity: a guide for health care organizations. IHI White Paper Cambridge. Massachusetts: Institute for Healthcare Improvement; 2016.

18. Sanchez NF, Rabatin J, Sanchez JP, et al. Medical students' ability to care for lesbian, gay, bisexual, and transgendered patients. Fam Med 2006;38(1):21.

19. Project Implicit. Project implicit. 2011. Available at: https://implicit.harvard.edu/implicit/index.jsp. Accessed July 16, 2019.

20. McDowell MJ, Berrahou IK. Learning to address implicit bias towards lgbtq patients: Case scenarios 2018, September.

21. Gay, Association LM. Guidelines for care of lesbian, gay, bisexual, and transgender patients. San Francisco (CA): Gay and Lesbian Medical Association; 2006.

22. Women CoHCfU. Committee Opinion no. 512: health care for transgender individuals. Obstet Gynecol 2011;118(6):1454.

23. Deutsch MB. Guidelines for the primary and gender-affirming care of transgender and gender nonbinary people. San Francisco (CA): University of California; 2016.

24. Hadland SE, Yehia BR, Makadon HJ. Caring for lesbian, gay, bisexual, transgender, and questioning youth in inclusive and affirmative environments. Pediatr Clin North Am 2016;63(6):955–69.

25. Tschurtz B, Burke A. The Joint Commission: advancing effective communication, cultural competence, and patient-and family-centered care for the lesbian, gay, bisexual, and transgender (LGBT) community: a field guide. In:2017.

26. Deutsch MB, Green J, Keatley J, et al. Electronic medical records and the transgender patient: recommendations from the World Professional Association for Transgender Health EMR Working Group. J Am Med Inform Assoc 2013;20(4): 700–3.

27. Donald C, Ehrenfeld J. The opportunity for medical systems to reduce health disparities among lesbian, gay, bisexual, transgender and intersex patients. J Med Syst 2015;39(11):1–7.

28. Cahill S, Makadon H. Sexual orientation and gender identity data collection in clinical settings and in electronic health records: A key to ending LGBT health disparities. LGBT Health 2014;1(1):34–41.

29. Shelton J, Poirier JM, Wheeler C, et al. Reversing erasure of youth and young adults who are lgbtq and access homelessness services: asking about sexual orientation, gender identity, and pronouns. Child Welfare 2018;96(2):1–28.

30. University of California San Francisco. Pronouns matter 2019. Available at: https://lgbt.ucsf.edu/pronounsmatter. Accessed November 4, 2019.

31. Logie CH, Lys CL, Dias L, et al. Automatic assumption of your gender, sexuality and sexual practices is also discrimination": Exploring sexual healthcare experiences and recommendations among sexually and gender diverse persons in Arctic Canada. Health Soc Care Community 2019;27(5):1204–13.

32. Annon JS. The PLISSIT model: A proposed conceptual scheme for the behavioral treatment of sexual problems. J Sex Educ Ther 1976;2(1):1–15.

33. Walker K, Arbour M, Waryold J. Educational strategies to help students provide respectful sexual and reproductive health care for lesbian, gay, bisexual, and transgender persons. J Midwifery Womens Health 2016;61(6):737–43.

Sexually Transmitted Infections in Pregnancy
An Update for Primary Care Providers

Melissa Glassford, DNP, FNP*, Melissa Davis, DNP, CNM, FNP,
Shelza Rivas, DNP, WHNP, AGPCNP

KEYWORDS

• Sexually transmitted infections • Pregnancy • Congenital infection

KEY POINTS

• Sexually transmitted infections are common and increasing in the United States; this includes the pregnant population and their unborn fetus.
• All pregnant women need to be screened for sexually transmitted infections at the initial obstetric visit as well as at 28 weeks if the patient is at increased risk of acquiring a sexually transmitted infection.
• Treatment of the most common sexually transmitted infections is outlined and discussed, including alternative regimens when applicable.

INTRODUCTION

Sexually transmitted infections (STIs) are among the most common acute infections worldwide. Infections are of particular importance in the health care of reproductive aged women, because STIs disproportionally affect women of reproductive age on both the national and the global level. It is well known that women are more vulnerable to long-term complications from STIs for a variety of reasons, including biological, social, and economic.[1,2] The long-term sequelae from untreated STIs include infertility, pelvic inflammatory disease (PID), and cervical cancer.[2] For pregnant women, the consequences of STIs can be both immediate and devastating. They range from ectopic pregnancy to preterm birth.[2] Mother-to-child transmission of STIs can result in neonatal death and disability.[2] As frontline clinicians, nurse practitioners and midwives should be well versed in the screening, early recognition, and treatment of STIs in reproductive aged women. The primary aim of this article is to highlight screening recommendations, treatment, safety, and when to refer when treating STIs in pregnant women.

Vanderbilt University School of Nursing, 461 21st Avenue South, Nashville, TN 37240, USA
* Corresponding author.
E-mail address: melissa.glassford@vanderbilt.edu

Nurs Clin N Am 55 (2020) 403–416
https://doi.org/10.1016/j.cnur.2020.06.004
0029-6465/20/© 2020 Elsevier Inc. All rights reserved.

nursing.theclinics.com

BACKGROUND

As a global phenomenon, STIs in pregnancy occur across the geographic spectrum, but some important regional distinctions exist. For example, the highest incidence and prevalence of syphilis occur in the African region, whereas chlamydia is estimated to be the highest in the regions of the Americas and Western Pacific.[3] However, although cases of syphilis have decreased worldwide, congenital syphilis has increased in the United States each year since 2013, sparking widespread public health concerns.[2–4] Syphilis is particularly concerning because more than half of pregnant women with untreated disease will have an adverse outcome, such as preterm birth, infant death, and even developmental disabilities in the surviving infants.[5] In the United States, chlamydia is the most common infection in pregnant women and has been found to significantly increase the risk of stillbirth and spontaneous abortion.[6]

Estimates of the prevalence of STIs in pregnancy can be difficult to obtain. Even STIs that are reportable may not include pregnancy status, further concealing the exact number of pregnant women affected and complicating epidemiology research.[7] A recent comprehensive survey of the Pregnancy Risk Assessment Monitoring System found that 3.3% of survey respondents indicated a diagnosis of one or more curable STIs during their most recent pregnancy.[7] Curable STIs include gonorrhea, chlamydia, syphilis, and trichomoniasis. Prevalence of chlamydia is thought to be around 3.5% of pregnant woman, and gonorrhea has about a 0.6% positivity rate, with younger age being a primary risk factor for both.[7]

Another source of data to examine STIs in pregnancy is individual state reporting of congenital syphilis in infants. In the most recent Centers for Disease Control and Prevention (CDC) report, there were 1306 reported cases of congenital syphilis in the United States in 2018 or 33.1% of 100,000 live births.[2] This data represents a greater than two-fold increase in the previous 10 years.[2] Neonatal herpes simplex virus (HSV) has also been trending upward, likely because of improved detection, but researchers examining Medicare and Medicaid data have found an overall incidence of 8.5 per 100,000 live births.[8] HSV infection rates demonstrate a variety of data regarding genital and orolabial infections. Although seroprevalance of HSV type 2 rates have remained stable, genital HSV type 1 lesion rates have increased in young adults, specifically in young childbearing women who are most likely to acquire HSV-1 or genital HSV-2 infections that later have implications in pregnancy.[9]

Another STI that affects pregnancy is trichomoniasis. It affects 2.3 million women between the ages of 14 and 49 years.[7] Epidemiologic data are difficult to obtain because trichomoniasis is not reportable. However, it is estimated that 3.2% of those with trichomoniasis are pregnant women.[10] Finally, the number of human immunodeficiency virus (HIV)-infected women who give birth is largely unknown, but the CDC does provide some data to inform the public. Older estimates from 2006 suggest that about 8500 women with HIV were giving birth in the United States annually but suggest that more recent estimates put that number at less than 5000.[11,12] In a sign of improved screening and treatment, rates of perinatal HIV infections have decreased by 41% between 2012 and 2016.[11]

There remains a considerable gap in the detection and treatment of STIs in women of childbearing age, particularly those of lower income. Disproportionally, younger women have much higher rates of gonorrhea and chlamydia.[7] STIs are significantly more common among women without health insurance before pregnancy and more common among non-Hispanic black women, unmarried women, and those with no college education.[7] Among all racial/ethnic groups, Hispanics had the lowest rate of health insurance in 2017 at 84% (CDC, 2018), placing them at higher risk for STIs before pregnancy. In examining the distribution of perinatal HIV, the CDC examined the demongraphics of 1814 children with diagnosed perinatal HIV in 2016.[11] Of these, approximately 63% were African American, 15% were Hispanic/Latino, and 11% were white, showing significant racial disparity that mirrors trends for nonpregnant women.[11]

Identifying the individual patients at risk for STIs and providing prompt screening and treatment should be a high priority for primary care providers. Early identification and intervention is particularly critical for women of childbearing age to reduce the risk and long-term impact of STI transmission to the fetus.

ANATOMY AND PHYSIOLOGY

The national and global prevalence of STIs in women demonstrates that both pregnant and nonpregnant women are at significant risk for contracting STIs compared with men. The nature of the female anatomy allows for infection transmission to more easily occur. The moist environment and thin tissue of the vagina allow easier penetration for bacteria and viruses.[1] Most STIs are asymptomatic in women, and oftentimes women confuse their symptoms as something else, such as yeast or bacterial vaginosis.[1] In the absence of easily identifiable symptoms, such as genital ulcers, STIs are more easily underdiagnosed and untreated.[1,2]

Pregnant women with STIs, specifically chlamydia, gonorrhea, syphilis, or HSV, pose a high risk of transmission from mother to baby during delivery. Mothers with active chlamydia and gonorrhea infections may cause eye and lung infections in their newborns.[10] Chlamydia and gonorrhea can also cause preterm labor, premature rupture of membranes (PROM), spontaneous abortion, premature birth, and low birth weight (LBW).[10] Congenital syphilis is caused by direct transmission of syphilis infection from mother to baby that can lead to serious and fatal newborn outcomes, such as premature birth, multisystem organ failure, still birth, and fetal death.[5,10,13] Last, the rate of HSV transmission from mother to baby is highest during delivery in mothers with active genital HSV infection and acquired genital HSV close to delivery.[8,10,14] Neonatal herpes simplex can also have serious complications, including HSV lesions, encephalitis, disseminated herpes infection, and fetal death.[10,15]

HIV can be transmitted from mother to baby during pregnancy, during delivery, and while breastfeeding.[11] Mothers who are not aware of their HIV-positive status, have a detectable viral load, and are not on viral suppressive therapy are most at risk for transmission to their baby during pregnancy.[11,16] A cesarean delivery is usually indicated to help prevent transmission of HIV from mother to infant.[11,16,17] Hepatitis C transmission rates are usually low in infected pregnant women at 10% likelihood of transmission unless the mother is also infected with HIV.[10] Newborns with hepatitis C are at increased risk for small for gestational age, premature birth, and LBW.[10]

SCREENING

Screening guidelines in the United States are robust in their support for universal screening of pregnant women. The US Preventative Services Task Force recommends screening all women for hepatitis B, HIV, and syphilis and also screening women aged 24 years and younger for gonorrhea and chlamydia.[18] The CDC has comprehensive screening guidelines for all STIs, which can be found in **Table 1**. Screening guidelines attempt to address the age disparity by recommending gonorrhea and chlamydia testing in all pregnant women aged 24 and younger and those at higher risk.[18] Guidelines address women who may have new sexual partners during pregnancy as well as partners with an STI. Furthermore, by taking an "opt-out" approach, health care

Table 1
Center for Disease Control and Prevention screening guidelines for all sexually transmitted infections

STI	CDC Recommendation
Evidence to support universal screening	
Chlamydia	First prenatal visit: Screen all pregnant women <25 y of age and older pregnant women at increased risk for infection Third trimester: Rescreen if <25 y of age or at continued high risk Risk factors: • New or multiple sex partners • Sex partner with concurrent partners • Sex partner who has a sexually transmitted disease (STD) NOTE: Pregnant women found to have chlamydial infection should have a test of cure 3 to 4 wk after treatment and then be retested within 3 mo
Gonorrhea	First prenatal visit: Screen all pregnant women <25 y of age and older pregnant women at increased risk for gonorrhea at first prenatal visit Third trimester: Rescreen for women at continued high risk Risk factors: • Living in a high-morbidity area • Previous or coexisting STI • New or multiple sex partners • Inconsistent condom use among persons not in mutually monogamous relationships • Exchanging sex for money or drugs
Syphilis	First prenatal visit: Screen all pregnant women. Early third trimester: Rescreen women • Who are at high risk for syphilis • Who live in areas with high numbers of syphilis cases, and • Who were not previously tested, or had a positive test in the first trimester
HIV	First prenatal visit: Screen all pregnant women Third trimester: Rescreen women at high risk for acquiring HIV infection
Hepatitis B (HBV)	First prenatal visit: Screen all pregnant women Third trimester: Test those who were not screened prenatally, those who engage in behaviors that put them at high risk for infection, and those with signs or symptoms of hepatitis at the time of admission to the hospital for delivery. Risk factors: • Having had more than 1 sex partner in the previous 6 mo • Evaluation or treatment of an STD • Recent or current injection-drug use • An HBsAg-positive sex partner
Hepatitis C (HCV)	First prenatal visit: Screen all pregnant women at increased risk Risk factors: • Past or current injection-drug use • Having received a blood transfusion before July 1992 • Receipt of unregulated tattoo • Long-term dialysis • Known exposure to HCV
Insufficient evidence to support universal screening	
Bacterial vaginosis (BV)	Evidence does not support routine screening for BV in asymptomatic pregnant women at high or low risk for preterm delivery

(continued on next page)

Table 1 (continued)	
STI	**CDC Recommendation**
Trichomoniasis	Evidence does not support routine screening for trichomoniasis in asymptomatic pregnant women
Herpes (HSV)	Evidence does not support routine HSV-2 serologic testing among asymptomatic pregnant women
Human papillomavirus (HPV)	There are no screening recommendations for HPV

From Center for Disease Control and Prevention C. STD Facts - STDs & Pregnancy Detailed Fact Sheet. Available at: https://www.cdc.gov/std/pregnancy/stdfact-pregnancy-detailed.htm. Published 2016. Accessed January 1, 2020. With permission.

providers can normalize screening, thereby eliminating the stigma often associated with STIs.[19] This approach allows clinicians to initiate STI screening for all pregnant women as an integral part of perinatal care.

INDIVIDUAL SEXUALLY TRANSMITTED INFECTIONS REVIEW
Trichomonas

Trichomonas, more commonly called "trich," is a common STI (**Table 2**). It is caused by a protozoa, *Trichomonas vaginalis*, and affects millions of people each year.[20] Because it is not a reportable infection and detection tests are often unreliable, the actual incidence of trichomonas is difficult to determine. It is speculated that trichomonas is the most commonly occurring nonviral STI.[20]

Transmission occurs by sexual contact, which transfers the protozoa via secretions to the urethra, vagina, and endocervix. Transmission to the fetus or a newborn during vaginal birth is rare. If it occurs, the newborn may experience fever and either genital or respiratory infection.[17]

Symptoms can include vaginal itching, irritation, lower abdominal pain, and malodorous yellow to green vaginal discharge. However, in more than 85% of cases in women, it is an asymptomatic infection.[20]

Risks associated with trichomonas infection during pregnancy include preterm birth, PROM, LBW babies, and uterine cramping.[17,21] In nonpregnant women, the main risks are transmission to other partners and personal discomfort. All women infected with trichomonas are at an increased risk of contracting HIV because of changes in vaginal pH resulting in altered vaginal flora, the inflammatory response related to trichomonas infection, and also because of microdamage to the vaginal walls caused by trichomonas, which results in a weaker barrier against HIV.[20,21]

Diagnosis is made through physical examination and laboratory testing. When performing a pelvic examination, the provider might notice a mildly irritated or slightly excoriated vulva, frothy yellow-green vaginal discharge, and occasionally a red, angry-appearing cervix (a "strawberry cervix").[17,20,21] Historically, a saline wet preparation was the main method used for diagnosis. The slide was considered positive when the presence of the pear-shaped, motile protozoan was identified. However, because of the insensitivity of the wet preparation, the CDC now recommends providers use more specific tests to decrease rates of false negatives.[21] Molecular detection tests, such as a polymerase chain reaction assay, are the recommended diagnostic test when available. Using these testing methods increases the sensitivity to 95% to 100% compared with the wet preparation's sensitivity of 51% to 65%.[21]

Table 2
Individual sexually transmitted infection review

STI	Recommended Treatment in Pregnant Women	Duration	Trimester Concerns	Alternatives	Other Considerations
Trichomonas	Metronidazole 2 g orally	One time/ single dose	Considered safe in every trimester; some providers wait until the second trimester out of an abundance of caution. Treatment should not be withheld in symptomatic women	Tinidazole: 2 g orally in a single dose	Avoid any products contacting alcohol for 24 h after taking metronidazole and for 72 h after taking tinidazole
Gonorrhea	Ceftriaxone 250 mg intramuscularly AND Azithromycin 1 g orally	Once Once	N/A	Only if unable to give Ceftriaxone: Cefixime (Suprax) 400 mg orally in a single dose AND azithromycin as described at left	Treat for both gonorrhea and chlamydia to reduce risk of antibiotic resistance and recurrent PID
Chlamydia	Azithromycin 1 g orally	Once	N/A	Amoxicillin 500 mg orally 3 times daily × 7 d	Can be treated as a single infection
HSV	Acyclovir 400 mg by mouth 3 times a day OR Acyclovir 200 mg by mouth 5 times a day OR Valacyclovir 1 g by mouth twice a day	7–10 d	N/A	N/A	Pregnant women with a history of genital HSV infection should begin prophylactic treatment at 36 wk' gestation and continue through delivery

HIV	Oral zidovudine	Throughout pregnancy	Throughout pregnancy	N/A	Managed by specialist care
Syphilis	Penicillin G 2.4 million units intramuscularly	Once	N/A	No alternatives during pregnancy; refer for desensitization if verified penicillin allergy	Dosing changes based on duration of infection
Hepatitis B & C					

Abbreviation: **N/A**, not applicable.
Data from Refs.[17,21]

Metronidazole (Flagyl) is the drug of choice in treating trichomonas.[21] Oral dosing is needed, because the gel preparation is not effective.[17] Multiple metaanalyses have found metronidazole to be safe in all stages of pregnancy, so there is no need to wait until the end of the first trimester to begin treatment.[20] Dosing is the same for pregnant and nonpregnant women: 2 g taken orally in one dose.[21] All women should be advised to avoid alcohol and alcohol-containing products for at least 24 hours after taking metronidazole. Partners need to be treated, even if they are asymptomatic.

Neisseria gonorrhoeae and Chlamydia trachomatis

Neisseria gonorrhoeae and Chlamydia trachomatis are often referred to together when discussing testing and treatment. The infections can accompany one another, and most of the available testing looks for both bacteria. Together, they are the 2 most common STIs reported to the health department and CDC, with Chlamydia being the most common.[17,22] Both are caused by small, gram-negative bacterium.[17,23,24]

Transmission of both gonorrhea and chlamydia occurs by sexual contact with infected secretions. It can be spread to the oropharynx and rectum, although genitourinary infection is the most common.[17]

Symptoms of chlamydia can include painful urination, vaginal discharge, and Bartholin gland infections. Gonorrhea infection can include these symptoms as well as bleeding between menstrual cycles.[17,25] However, most chlamydia and gonorrheal infections are asymptomatic, which is why universal screening is so critical.[17,24]

Risks of chlamydial and gonococcal infection include damage to the female reproductive system. If left untreated, the bacteria can ascend higher into the reproductive tract and cause PID, which can lead to scarring in the uterus and fallopian tubes and increase the likelihood of infertility, and ectopic pregnancy in the future.[17] In pregnant women, it can lead to uterine cramping, early delivery, PROM, low neonatal birth weight, stillbirth, and infections in the neonate.[2]

Other risks of gonorrhea and chlamydia are specific to the neonate. Chlamydia can cause pneumonia, whereas both gonorrhea and chlamydia can lead to an eye infection called ophthalmia neonatorum.[2,24,26] The eye infection is serious and can result in blindness. This adverse outcome has led to the recommendation that all pregnant women be screened for gonorrhea and chlamydia infection, and that all neonates receive prophylactic erythromycin eye ointment at birth.[24,26]

Diagnosis of both chlamydia and gonorrhea is made through the use of nucleic acid amplification testing and can be performed on a dirty-catch urine specimen or by collecting a swab specimen from the vagina or endocervix.[24] The physical examination may be unremarkable in early infection. In later infection, there may be mucopurulent vaginal or urethral discharge and/or the presence of cervical motion tenderness. Once the infection has progressed to PID, the physical examination becomes more remarkable with extreme cervical motion tenderness, abdominal pain, rebound tenderness, and fever.[27] Women with PID may experience pain with walking, appear stooped, and shuffle their feet, hence the common phrase, PID shuffle, although this is a more rare presentation.[28]

Medication dosing and safety

For chlamydia treatment during pregnancy, the CDC recommends Azithromycin (Zithromax) 1 g in a single dose as first-line treatment with an alternative regimen of Amoxicillin 500 mg by mouth 3 times daily for 7 days.[24] For gonorrhea treatment during pregnancy, current guidelines recommend treating gonorrhea with Ceftriaxone (Rocephin) 250 mg intramuscularly PLUS Azithromycin 1 g in a single dose.[23] It has been a long-standing recommendation to treat for both gonorrhea and chlamydia when treating for gonorrhea because of the frequency of the infections occurring together, as well as to improve efficacy of treatment and reduce potential for resistance to cephalosporins.[23,24,29] Pregnant women need a test of cure 3 to 4 weeks after completing treatment of either or both infections.[17,24]

Herpes Simplex Virus

HSV can present as type 1 or 2. Historically, type 1 was thought to only affect the mouth and nose, but it is now known that both types can cause genital lesions.[14]

Transmission is via contact and can be spread by kissing as well as through sexual contact. Type 1 is typically contracted in childhood through oral contact, but it can also be transmitted to the genitals via orogenital contact. Type 2 is classically known as genital herpes and can be spread by sexual contact. Both types can be transmitted even if the infected individual has no symptoms or active lesions; this is called viral shedding. Vertical transmission between mother and fetus can occur, although the greatest transmission risk to baby is at birth via contact with HSV in maternal secretions.[14,15,17]

Symptoms include painful vesicular lesions occurring on the mouth, perineum, vulva, or anus. The discomfort is typically disproportionate to the size of the lesion.[17] A speculum examination is not necessary and may be very painful for the woman. Before outbreak of lesions, the woman may experience vague symptoms, such as myalgias, fever, headaches, and general malaise. She may also experience a prodromal tingling or burning of the skin before eruption of lesions.[17]

Risks of HSV are mainly related to vertical transmission to the baby.[14] A primary outbreak is much more likely to cause infection in the fetus, although secondary outbreaks can also cause infection. The main risk associated with HSV during pregnancy, other than discomfort to the woman, is that of transmission to the neonate during birth. Neonatal HSV infection can be serious and even life-threatening and can include respiratory distress, jaundice, irritability, and seizures.[2,17]

When the pregnant woman with a history of genital herpes presents in labor, she will need a speculum examination and visualization of the labia and vulva before birth. If there are active genital lesions present, or if she is having prodromal symptoms of an impending outbreak, delivery by cesarean section is recommended.[17]

Diagnosis can be made by physical examination and confirmed by viral and serologic testing. A viral culture can be sent using the exudate from an active lesion, but this is not very sensitive, especially if the lesion is already crusted over.[17] Blood testing to confirm diagnosis and reveal the subtype is recommended by the CDC.[30] Although the types are treated the same, HSV-2 can be more infectious and more likely to shed in the absence of lesions.[30]

An oral antiviral is recommended for HSV outbreaks. Acyclovir (Zovirax) 400 mg by mouth 3 times a day for 7 to 10 days or Valacyclovir (Valtrex) 1 g by mouth twice a day for 7 to 10 days is commonly used.[30] Women with severe initial outbreaks during pregnancy may need to be evaluated for intravenous acyclovir. Pregnant women with a history of genital HSV need to begin acyclovir prophylaxis at 36 weeks' gestation to minimize the risk of active lesions at the time of labor and birth.[17]

Human Immunodeficiency Virus

HIV is an RNA retrovirus that eventually affects the body's CD4 cells, which are critical for the immune response. As of 2016, there were 1.1 million adults in the United States living with HIV. Of that number, almost 14% are unaware of their HIV status.[31]

Transmission occurs through sexual contact. Women with other STIs, including herpes, gonorrhea, chlamydia, or others resulting in lesions in the genital tract, are at higher risk of contracting HIV.[2] Also, sexual practices that cause more damage to the vaginal or rectal mucosa can increase a woman's risk of HIV infection.[17,31]

Symptoms can be vague and include infectious mononucleosis-like symptoms, such as fever, body aches, skin rash, diarrhea, nausea, sore throat, and headache. These symptoms typically occur within a few weeks of infection. After this period of general malaise, the infection becomes asymptomatic for up to 8 years.[17,32] Although asymptomatic, the virus is still replicating and multiplying until it begins to affect the carrier's CD4 cells. Once the CD4 cell count decreases below a certain point, symptoms of AIDS begin to show. These symptoms can include weight loss, fever, cough, shortness of breath, and more severe illnesses than one would expect for the person's age and history.[17,32]

Risks during pregnancy are mostly related to the risk of neonatal transmission. Pregnancy itself does not hasten the progression from HIV infection to AIDS.[32] The risk of transmission to baby can be significantly reduced by appropriate care and treatment during pregnancy as well as a planned delivery at 38 weeks. Delivery type is determined by CD4 counts and viral load determination. Women with elevated viral loads need to be delivered by cesarean section to minimize exposure. If a vaginal birth is planned, physiologic birth is recommended with special regards to avoidance of fetal scalp electrodes, episiotomies, and operative vaginal deliveries.[17] HIV can be transmitted to the neonate via breast milk. Therefore, women living with HIV should not breastfeed as long as there is a safe feeding alternative, such as formula mixed with clean water.[33]

Diagnosis is made by serologic testing for antibodies to HIV-1 and HIV-2, ideally, a combination HIV-1/HIV-2 antigen/antibody immunoassay. If this test is reactive, then a confirmatory HIV-1/HIV-2 antibody differentiation test, such as the Western blot, is performed.[32] All pregnant women need to be screened early in pregnancy as well as in the third trimester before 36 weeks.[16]

Treatment of HIV during pregnancy is managed by specialists and is dependent on multiple factors. Medication regimens are customized based on maternal health status, comorbid conditions, and disease processes.[17,34] Antiviral medications, such as oral zidovudine (AZT, Retrovir), are used during pregnancy to decrease the risk of vertical transmission as well as in the neonate soon after birth.[34]

Syphilis

Syphilis is an infection caused by a spiral-shaped spirochete called *Treponema pallidum*.[35] In 2017, there were 30,644 cases of primary or secondary syphilis in the United States, equivalent to 9.5 cases per 100,000 people.[36] Syphilis can be difficult to detect because it can mimic other infections or have no symptoms at all until the infection is advanced.[17] Syphilis infection, including congenital infection, has been on the rise over the past 10 years.[35,37]

Transmission occurs by vaginal, oral, or anal sexual contact. Condoms can reduce transmission rates, but only if lesions are completely covered by the condom.[17] The characteristic chancre associated with early syphilis is highly contagious while present, but often goes unnoticed. Vertical transmission occurs when a pregnant woman transmits the infection to the unborn fetus via the placenta or during birth.[17,37]

Symptoms are frequently absent. In the primary phase, a chancre will appear at the site of infection within about 3 weeks from exposure. The lone chancre is painless, highly contagious, and often goes unnoticed, especially if it is in the vagina or rectum.[17] Characteristics of the chancre include a flat base and red, raised border, with an ulcerated middle.[17,37] The chancre typically resolves within 2 to 8 weeks. Secondary syphilis marks the change from localized infection to systemic infection, usually within 4 to 10 weeks after infection. The hallmark symptom of this phase is a rash that occurs on the trunk, palms of hands, and soles of the feet.[17] Other symptoms can occur, but are vague and nonspecific. These symptoms include low-grade fever, malaise, headache, sore throat, lack of appetite, and generalized lymphadenopathy. Condyloma are flat, wartlike lesions that can most commonly develop and be found in body folds, such as the vulva and around the anus.[17] The third stage of syphilis, called tertiary syphilis, is rare. It can develop up to 30 years after the initial infection and can lead to neurologic and/or cardiovascular disease.[17]

Syphilis crosses the placenta after about 9 weeks' gestation, whereas congenital infection typically occurs between 16 and 28 weeks' gestation.[17] Studies suggest that in women with untreated syphilis during pregnancy, up to 40% will end in neonatal deaths.[5] Others are at risk for stillbirth, congenital malformations, congenital infection, LBW, and preterm birth.[5,17,37]

Diagnosis is usually made serologically by non-treponemal testing followed by a treponemal-specific confirmatory test. Nontreponemal tests, such as the Venereal Disease Research Laboratory (VRDL) or the rapid plasma regain (RPR) card test, are nonspecific antibody tests.[37] If one of these tests is positive, a confirmation treponemal-specific test is performed. If the test is negative, this likely represents a false positive on the initial nontreponemal test. Women with a false positive test should have repeat testing performed after 4 weeks. If the second treponemal test is positive, the patient has either active or past infection with syphilis. Women who have successfully been treated do not need further management. Women who do not have evidence of treatment will need staging and treatment. When tracking titers for treatment efficacy, the same test (either the VRDL or the RPR) needs to be used for comparison purposes.[35,37,38] All pregnant women with either a positive or a false positive test should be evaluated for signs and symptoms of syphilis, testing repeated where indicated, and have close follow-up.[35]

Penicillin is the only known effective drug for the treatment of syphilis infection. Dosing is contingent on the stage of syphilis and duration of infection. In general, penicillin G 2.4 million units intramuscularly in a single dose is the recommendation. If the pregnant woman is allergic to penicillin, inpatient desensitization is recommended. Any patient with advanced syphilis needs to be referred for specialty care.[17,35,37]

Zika Virus

Zika is a relatively new virus and is transmitted to humans by an infected mosquito. However, once a person contracts the virus from the mosquito, it can be spread by sexual contact. Most people with Zika are asymptomatic. However, symptoms of Zika virus can include fever, headache, arthralgias, muscle aches, and rash, but the person infected can be contagious before showing symptoms as well as after symptoms have resolved.[39,40] The virus has been identified in South and Central America, Africa, and Asia, although infected persons have carried the virus further.[41] Pregnant women traveling to an area known to be high risk for Zika or those with a partner traveling to those areas should exercise caution. All parties should protect themselves from mosquito bites, and condoms should be worn or abstinence observed for the duration of pregnancy.[40] Zika conveys significant risk to the fetus/neonate, including stillbirth, eye abnormalities, growth restriction, microcephaly, and other brain defects.[17,40] When discussing Zika virus, it is important that primary care providers consult the CDC for the most up-to-date recommendations and consult specialists for guidance. Currently, there is no vaccine, nor is there treatment or antiviral prophylaxis for this virus.[17,40]

SUMMARY

STIs pose significant health risks to women and infants across the United States. Untreated, STIs pose a considerable economic burden during labor and delivery as well as long-term care on the child owing to disability. Any health care provider who may see women of childbearing age, from adolescence onward, should be well versed in the screening recommendations and necessity of prompt treatment. A key takeaway from this article is that most STIs are asymptomatic, particularly early in the course of infection. Relying on patients to present with obvious symptoms will not adequately address the public health concerns of untreated STIs and transmission to the fetus. Understanding of the disparities in race, economic, insurance status, and age should be combined with robust universal screening, guideline adherence, and protection of women and infants in the United States.

DISCLOSURE

The authors have nothing to disclose.

REFERENCES

1. Cdc.gov. 10 Ways Stds Impact Women Differently From Men. [online] 2011. Available at: https://www.cdc.gov/std/health-disparities/STDs-Women-042011.pdf. Accessed July 15, 2020.
2. Center for Disease Control and Prevention. STDs in women and infants - 2018 sexually transmitted diseases surveillance. 2019. Available at: https://www.cdc.gov/std/stats18/womenandinf.htm. Accessed December 28, 2019.
3. Newman L, Rowley J, Vander Hoorn S, et al. Global estimates of the prevalence and incidence of four curable sexually transmitted infections in 2012 based on systematic review and global reporting. PLoS One 2015;10(12):e0143304. Meng Z, ed.
4. Bachmann LH. A devastating surge in congenital syphilis: how can we stop it? Medscape. 2019. Available at: https://www.medscape.com/viewarticle/907183?src=par_cdc_stm_mscpedt&faf=1. Accessed January 1, 2020.
5. Gomez GB, Kamb ML, Newman LM, et al. Systematic reviews untreated maternal syphilis and adverse outcomes of pregnancy: a systematic review and meta-analysis. Bull World Heal Organ 2013;91:217–26.
6. Tang W, Mao J, Li KT, et al. Pregnancy and fertility-related adverse outcomes associated with Chlamydia trachomatis infection: a global systematic review and meta-analysis. Sex Transm Infect 2019. https://doi.org/10.1136/SEXTRANS-2019-053999.
7. Williams CL, Harrison LL, Llata E, et al. Sexually transmitted diseases among pregnant women: 5 states, United States, 2009-2011. Matern Child Health J 2018;22(4):538–45.
8. Donda K, Sharma M, Amponsah JK, et al. Trends in the incidence, mortality, and cost of neonatal herpes simplex virus hospitalizations in the United States from 2003 to 2014. J Perinatol 2019;39(5):697–707.
9. Centers for Disease Control and Prevention. Sexually Transmitted Disease Surveillance 2018. Atlanta: U.S. Department of Health and Human Services; 2019.
10. Center for Disease Control and Prevention C. STD facts - STDs & pregnancy detailed fact sheet. 2016. Available at: https://www.cdc.gov/std/pregnancy/stdfact-pregnancy-detailed.htm. Accessed January 1, 2020.

11. Center for Disease Control and Prevention C. Pregnant women, infants, and children | gender | HIV by group | HIV/AIDS | CDC. 2012. Available at: https://www.cdc.gov/hiv/group/gender/pregnantwomen/index.html. Accessed January 1, 2020.

12. Fontenot HB, George ER. Sexually transmitted infections in pregnancy. Nurs Womens Health 2014;18(1):67–72.

13. Korenromp EL, Rowley J, Alonso M, et al. Global burden of maternal and congenital syphilis and associated adverse birth outcomes—estimates for 2016 and progress since 2012. PLoS One 2019;14(2):e0211720. Vellakkal S, ed.

14. James SH, Sheffield JS, Kimberlin DW. Mother-to-child transmission of herpes simplex virus. J Pediatr Infect Dis Soc 2014;3(SUPPL1). https://doi.org/10.1093/jpids/piu050.

15. Stephenson-Famy A, Gardella C. Herpes simplex virus infection during pregnancy. Obstet Gynecol Clin North Am 2014;41(4):601–14.

16. American College of Obstetrics and Gynecology. ACOG Committee Opinion No. 752 summary: prenatal and perinatal human immunodeficiency virus testing. Obstet Gynecol 2018;132(3):805–6.

17. King TL, Brucker MC, Jevitt C, et al. (Nurse-midwife). Varney's midwifery (6th edition). Burlington (MA): Jones & Bartlett Learning; 2019.

18. Lee KC, Ngo-Metzger Q, Wolff T, et al. Sexually Transmitted Infections: Recommendations from the U.S. Preventive Services Task Force. Am Fam Physician 2016;94(11):907–15.

19. Selph SS, Bougatsos C, Dana T, et al. Screening for HIV infection in pregnant women: updated evidence report and systematic review for the US Preventive Services Task Force. JAMA 2019;321(23):2349–60.

20. Kissinger P. Epidemiology and treatment of trichomoniasis. Curr Infect Dis Rep 2015;17(6):31.

21. Center for Disease Control and Prevention. Trichomoniasis - 2015 STD Treatment Guidelines. 2015. Available at: https://www.cdc.gov/std/tg2015/trichomoniasis.htm. Accessed December 30, 2019.

22. Centers for Disease Control and Prevention. Sexually Transmitted Disease Surveillance 2013. Atlanta: U.S. Department of Health and Human Services; 2014.

23. Center for Disease Control and Prevention C. Gonococcal infections - 2015 STD Treatment Guidelines. 2015. Available at: https://www.cdc.gov/std/tg2015/gonorrhea.htm. Accessed January 1, 2020.

24. Center for Disease Control and Prevention C. Chlamydial infections - 2015 STD Treatment Guidelines. 2015. Available at: https://www.cdc.gov/std/tg2015/chlamydia.htm. Accessed December 30, 2019.

25. Center for Disease Control and Prevention. STD facts - Gonorrhea. 2014. Available at: https://www.cdc.gov/std/gonorrhea/stdfact-gonorrhea.htm. Accessed December 30, 2019.

26. Vainder M, Kives S, Yudin MH. Screening for gonorrhea and chlamydia in pregnancy: room for improvement. J Obstet Gynaecol Can 2019;41(9):1289–94.

27. Mitchell C, Prabhu M. Pelvic inflammatory disease: current concepts in pathogenesis, diagnosis and treatment. Infect Dis Clin North Am 2013;27(4):793–809.

28. Trent M. Pelvic inflammatory disease. Pediatr Rev 2013;34(4):163–72.

29. Ros ST. What is new in sexually transmitted infections? Obstet Gynecol 2018;131(5):928–9.

30. Center for Disease Control and Prevention C. Genital HSV infections - 2015 STD Treatment Guidelines. 2015. Available at: https://www.cdc.gov/std/tg2015/herpes.htm. Accessed January 1, 2020.

31. Centers for Disease Control and Prevention. Estimated HIV incidence and prevalence in the United States, 2010–2015. HIV Surveillance Supplemental Report 2018;23(No. 1). Published March 2018. Available at: http://www.cdc.gov/hiv/library/reports/hiv-surveillance.html. Accessed July 15, 2020.

32. Center for Disease Control and Prevention C. HIV infection: detection, counseling, and referral - 2015 STD Treatment Guidelines. 2015. Available at: https://www.cdc.gov/std/tg2015/hiv.htm. Accessed January 1, 2020.

33. American Academy of Pediatrics. Human Immunodeficiency Virus Infection 111. In: Kimberlin DW, Brady MT, Jackson MA, et al, editors. Red Book: 2018 Report of the Committee on Infectious Diseases. American Academy of Pediatrics; 2018. p. 459–76.

34. Panel on Treatment of Pregnant Women with HIV Infection and Prevention of Perinatal Transmission. Recommendations for Use of Antiretroviral Drugs in Transmission in the United States. Available at: http://aidsinfo.nih.gov/contentfiles/lvguidelines/PerinatalGL.pdf. Accessed July 15, 2020.

35. Center for Disease Control and Prevention C. Syphilis - 2015 STD Treatment Guidelines. 2015. Available at: https://www.cdc.gov/std/tg2015/syphilis.htm. Accessed December 30, 2019.

36. Center for Disease Control and Prevention C. Syphilis - 2017 Sexually Transmitted Diseases Surveillance. 2017. Available at: https://www.cdc.gov/std/stats17/syphilis.htm. Accessed December 30, 2019.

37. Tsimis ME, Sheffield JS. Update on syphilis and pregnancy. Birth Defect Res 2017;109(5):347–52.

38. Curry SJ, Krist AH, Owens DK, et al. Screening for syphilis infection in pregnant women. JAMA 2018;320(9):911.

39. Moreira J, Peixoto TM, Siqueira AM, et al. Sexually acquired Zika virus: a systematic review. Clin Microbiol Infect 2017;23(5):296–305.

40. Center for Disease Control and Prevention. Clinical evaluation & disease | Zika virus | CDC. 2019. Available at: https://www.cdc.gov/zika/hc-providers/preparing-for-zika/clinicalevaluationdisease.html. Accessed January 1, 2020.

41. Center for Disease Control and Prevention. Overview | Zika virus | CDC. 2019. Available at: https://www.cdc.gov/zika/about/overview.html. Accessed January 1, 2020.

Update on Clinical Practice Guidelines for Human Immunodeficiency Virus

Courtney J. Pitts, DNP, MPH, FNP-BC

KEYWORDS

- Human immunodeficiency virus • Pathophysiology • Antiretroviral therapy
- Pregnancy • Adults • Adolescents • Children

KEY POINTS

- The management of human immunodeficiency virus has evolved since the first reported case.
- Prevention efforts should account for social norms, structural barriers, and individual characteristics.
- Antiretroviral therapy is a treatment as prevention strategy because it prevents HIV transmission and is efficient at viral suppression.
- It is important for health care professionals to be knowledgeable of clinical practice guidelines for HIV management in adults, children, and pregnant women.

INTRODUCTION

It has been more than 38 years since the first reported case of human immunodeficiency virus (HIV). Over this period of time, there has been an evolution in the care, management, and survival of those living with HIV and acquired immunodeficiency syndrome (AIDS). Such changes in the approach to the management and prevention of HIV have resulted in a plateau in the number of new diagnoses within recent years within the United States.[1] According to the Centers for Disease Control and Prevention (CDC), more than 38,000 persons were diagnosed with HIV in 2017, with the largest subpopulation affected being men who have sex with men.[2] The largest racial and age groups affected were black/African American and those between 25 years old and 34 years old, respectively.[2] As of 2016, there were more than 1 million people living with HIV (PLWH) in the United States.[1] This speaks volumes to the screening, diagnosis, retention, and viral suppression efforts of health care providers who care for PLWH. It is critical that health care providers are knowledgeable of the pathophysiology of HIV, related risk factors, and transmission routes to be able to effectively care

Vanderbilt University School of Nursing, 461 21st Avenue South, Nashville, TN 37240, USA
E-mail address: courtney.j.pitts@vanderbilt.edu

Nurs Clin N Am 55 (2020) 417–427
https://doi.org/10.1016/j.cnur.2020.06.005
0029-6465/20/© 2020 Elsevier Inc. All rights reserved.
nursing.theclinics.com

for PLWH. With this knowledge, health care providers will be equipped with the necessary tools to treat PLWH holistically.

PATHOPHYSIOLOGY

The pathophysiologic process of HIV includes 5 stages: binding and entry, reverse transcriptase, integration, protein synthesis, and budding. After HIV has been transmitted to a susceptible host, the HIV virion binds to glycoproteins that facilitate its attachment to the CD4$^+$ receptors and CCR5 coreceptors of the susceptible cell. Once attached, the glycoproteins initiate fusion between the viral envelope and the cell's plasma membrane. This allows the core of the virus to enter the cytoplasm, where it is uncoated and releases viral RNA. The reverse transcription process then converts the RNA to DNA provirus. The DNA provirus migrates into the nucleus of the host cell, where it integrates into the host cell's DNA. The virus may remain latent or become activated. If activated, the provirus becomes viral protein precursors that are synthesized into smaller proteins. These proteins assemble the viral RNA into new mature virions that bud from the cell and move to other host cells within the body.

TYPES OF HUMAN IMMUNODEFICIENCY VIRUS

There are 2 types of HIV, HIV-1 and HIV-2. HIV-1 is found more commonly worldwide.[3] HIV-2 is found predominantly in Western African. HIV-2 rarely is seen in the United States unless the person is originally from Western Africa. Although both types of HIV are transmitted through the same routes and are associated with the same opportunistic infections, there are some differences.[3] Both types of HIV are biologically similar but HIV-1 has proved to have reduced virulence, with a slower rate of CD4 T-cell decline. HIV-2 is not as easily transmittable as HIV-1. The period between the initial infection and the actual occurrence of the illness is longer with HIV-2, making it less pathogenic.[3] HIV-1 has an easier perinatal transmission. With HIV-2, infants may be breastfed in the absence of interventions because there is a 0% to 5% transmission rate. Laboratory testing can be performed to confirm the type of HIV if there is a suspicion that a person in the United States has HIV-2.

STAGES OF HUMAN IMMUNODEFICIENCY VIRUS

There are 3 clinical stages of HIV. Stage 1 is the acute HIV infection that typically occurs 2 weeks to 4 weeks after infection.[4] This stage manifests as an acute retroviral syndrome, because it often resembles hallmark symptoms of other common viruses (influenza, infectious mononucleosis, and so forth) that may last a few weeks.[4,5] At this time, a person is highly infectious and typically has a viral load in the millions. This then is followed by seroconversion in which antibodies are being developed. This process may take up to 3 months. The antibodies being developed are indicative of infection and can be confirmed with laboratory testing. The second stage is known as the clinical latency or HIV dormancy stage.[4,5] During this stage, a person infected with HIV is asymptomatic although HIV replication continues to occur at very low levels, making them infectious. This stage can last anywhere from 3 months to decades, depending on the presence of antiretroviral therapy (ART). If untreated, the CD4 cell count decreases as the HIV viral load increases, resulting in more pronounced symptoms, transitioning the person to stage 3. Stage 2 is characterized by a significantly compromised immune system, clinical symptoms, and even severe illnesses, known as opportunistic infections (**Box 1**).[6] This is the stage in which a person has AIDS. A person may present clinically with symptoms, including, but not limited to,

Box 1
Human immunodeficiency virus–related opportunistic infections
Candidiasis (thrush) of bronchi, trachea, esophagus, or lungs
Coccidioidomycosis
Cryptococcosis
Cryptosporidiosis
Cytomegalovirus, in particular retinitis
Encephalopathy
Herpes simplex virus
Histoplasmosis
Invasive cervical cancer
Isosporiasis
Kaposi sarcoma
Lymphoma, various forms
Mycobacterium avium complex
Pneumocystis carinii pneumonia
Pneumonia, recurrent
Progressive multifocal leukoencephalopathy
Salmonella
Toxoplasmosis
Tuberculosis
Wasting syndrome
Adapted from Centers for Disease Control and Prevention. Revised surveillance case definition for HIV infection – United States, 2014. Morbidity and Mortality Weekly Report: Recommendations and reports, 63 (RR03); 1 – 10. Available at https://www.cdc.gov/mmwr/preview/mmwrhtml/rr6303a1.htm. Accessed December 30, 2019. With permission.

fever, chills, sweating, swollen lymph nodes, and unexplained weight loss. AIDS is diagnosed clinically when there are changes in the CD4 cell count or in the presence of certain opportunistic infections (**Table 1**).[4–7] If a person in stage 3 is untreated, it can lead to death.

RISK FACTORS

HIV is transmitted primarily from person to person via body fluids (**Box 2**).[8] These body fluids typically are exchanged through unprotected sexual intercourse or the use of injectable drug equipment.[8] There are predisposing factors that increase the likelihood of a person acquiring HIV:

- Engaging in unprotected vaginal, anal, or oral sex
- Having untreated sexually transmitted infections (STIs)
- Sharing contaminated syringes and other injectable equipment with someone who has HIV
- Engaging in active substance abuse
- Avoiding management of mental conditions

Table 1
Case definition of human immunodeficiency virus and acquired immunodeficiency syndrome in adolescents and adults

| Stage[a] | Laboratory Evidence | |
	CD4 Cell Count	CD4 Percentage
1	≥500 cells/μL	≥26
2	200–499 cells/μL	14–25
3	<200 cells/μL	<14

[a] Staging is based on the CD4 cell count. The CD4 percentage is considered when the CD4 cell count is not available. In the presence of an opportunistic infection, it is stage 3 regardless of CD4 cell count or percentage. Staging differs for those less than 6 y of age.
Data from Refs.[4–7]

- Being pregnant while not receiving ART
- Receiving blood transfusions or having medical procedures with unsterile equipment[8,9]

Understanding these risk factors, their prevalence within a particular geographic setting, and the prevalence of HIV in that same geographic setting is vital to HIV prevention efforts.

PREVENTION EFFORTS

For the past couple decades, prevention efforts have targeted social norms, structural barriers, and individual characteristics that were determined to be risk factors for HIV transmission through sex or blood in specific geographic settings.[10,11] Efforts targeting social norms focused on culture, community, socioeconomic status, and geographic location.[11] To address structural barriers, prevention efforts focused on gender inequalities, stigma, racism, violence, economic inequality, poverty, and criminalization.[10,11] Prevention efforts on the individual level targeted issues related to age, gender, identity, and profession.[11] Overall, the promotion of condom use, partner reduction or abstinence, and needle exchange programs were the most consistent initiatives across geographic settings that accounted for these risk factors at some level.[10] Coupled with HIV treatment, these efforts have been critical to the decline of HIV incidence worldwide.

Box 2
Body fluids that transmit human immunodeficiency virus

Blood

Breast milk

Preseminal fluid

Rectal fluids

Semen

Vaginal fluids

From AIDSinfo. HIV/AIDS: The basics. 2019. Available at https://aidsinfo.nih.gov/understanding-hiv-aids/fact-sheets/19/45/hiv-aids–the-basics. Accessed on December 30, 2019. With permission.

Pharmacologically, the availability of medication to prevent HIV has transitioned. For more than 20 years, there has been ART, known as postexposure prophylaxis, available to treat occupational and nonoccupational exposures to HIV for persons who were HIV negative.[12] This regimen typically is initiated within 72 hours of exposure but has proved more effective if initiated within 36 hours.[12,13] More recently, the availability of a pre-exposure prophylaxis (PrEP) has elevated prevention efforts as work continues to ensue to stabilize HIV incidence and end the HIV/AIDS epidemic. PrEP is a 1-pill-a-day oral regimen that can be used among those at highest risk to prevent HIV acquisition.[14] To date, there are 2 regimens approved for prescription as PrEP. Although there continue to be pharmacologic advances, they do not guarantee PrEP as a lone preventive effort because accessibility, cost, availability, and risk perception are barriers to its effectiveness.[14] Therefore, it is of utter importance that prevention efforts continue to couple PrEP with initiatives targeting individual characteristics, social norms, and structural barriers.

Antiretroviral Therapy as Prevention

According to the CDC, there are 4 goals when managing PLWH—diagnosis, establishment of care, retention in care, and lastly viral suppression.[15] This means that adequate screening has to take place to find those who are undiagnosed. Once diagnosed, these persons must establish care for HIV management within 1 month.[15] After care is established, efforts are made to retain them in care and to subsequently suppress their virus by treating them with ART.[15] The last goal is critical to the prevention of HIV, commonly known as a treatment as prevention strategy. Adherence to effective ART regimens leads to viral suppression. Viral suppression is defined as maintaining HIV RNA levels less than 200 copies/mL, which can prevent transmission of the virus to a new host.[16]

There currently are 7 drug classes of ART: nucleoside reverse transcriptase inhibitors (NRTIs), non-NRTI (NNRTIs), protease inhibitors (PIs), integrase inhibitors (INSTIs), entry inhibitors, fusion inhibitors, and a CD4 T-lymphocyte postattachment inhibitor.[17] Cobicistat and ritonavir serve as pharmacokinetic enhancers, or boosters, to improve the effectiveness of PIs and the INSTI elvitegravir.[17] Each drug class is indicative of the point at which it stops the HIV replication pathophysiologic process. NRTIs and NNRTIs halt the reverse transcriptase process.[18] PIs prevent the protein synthesis process that produces new virions. INSTIs halt integration of the HIV DNA into the host cell's DNA. Entry or fusion inhibitors prevent the HIV virion from gaining entry into the host cell by blocking its ability to binding to the cell's receptors and coreceptors.[18] ART regimens are composed of 2 or 3 drugs from 2 different drug classes to effectively halt the HIV replication in at least 2 of its 5 stages.[16,17] Currently, there are more than 30 pharmacologic agents approved by the US Food and Drug Administration as either individual or coformulated regimens for ART.

Guidelines for First-Line Regimens for Adolescents and Adults

Advances in technology have resulted in the availability of newer antiretroviral drugs with lower pill burden, safer drug profiles, and increased durability. The availability of these new medications are reflected in the most up-to-date guidelines for initial therapy as recommended by the Department of Health and Human Services (DHHS) or the International Antiviral Society–USA (IAS-USA) on first-line regimens for the treatment and viral suppression of HIV (**Table 2**).[16,17] Although there are some similarities in the recommendations, there also are some differences. The DHHS guidelines recommends 5 options for initial therapy, with 1 of them a 2-drug, 2-drug class option. This differs from the traditional 3-drug, 2-class options presented

Table 2
First-line antiretroviral therapy regimen recommendations for adults and adolescents

Department of Health and Human Services	International Antiviral Society–USA

• Bictegravir/TAF/emtricitabine
• Dolutegravir/abacavir/lamivudine[a,d]
• Dolutegravir + emtricitabine
  or lamivudine + TAF or TDF[b,d]
• Dolutegravir/lamivudine[c,d]
• Raltegravir + emtricitabine
  or lamivudine + TAF or TDF
	• Bictegravir/TAF/emtricitabine
	• Dolutegravir/abacavir/lamivudine[a,d]
	• Dolutegravir +TAF or emtricitabine[d]

[a] HLA-B*5701 must be negative when considering the use of abacavir. Cannot have chronic hepatitis B virus coinfection. Consider a TDF-based regimen for those with or at risk of cardiovascular disease.
[b] TAF and TDF are virologically similar. TAF, however, has a safer profile because it has fewer bone and kidney toxicities compared with TDF. TDF is known to be associated with lower lipid levels.
[c] Individual cannot have an HIV RNA greater than 500,000 copies/mL, chronic hepatitis B virus coinfection, or, in the absence of HIV, genotypic resistance testing or hepatitis B testing.
[d] Initiation of dolutegravir in women of childbearing age raises concerns due to possible teratogenic effects when initiated before conception.
Data from Panel on antiretroviral guidelines for adults and adolescents. Guidelines for the use of antiretroviral agents in adults and adolescents with HIV. 2019. Department of Health and Human Services. Available at http://www.aidsinfo.nih.gov/ContentFiles/AdultandAdolescentGL.pdf. Accessed on January 1, 2020. And Saag, M., Benson, C., Gandhi, R., and et al. Antiretroviral Drugs for Treatment and Prevention of HIV Infection in Adults 2018 Recommendations of the International Antiviral Society–USA Panel. JAMA. 2018; 320(4):379-396.

by the IAS-USA. The DHHS guidelines also offers more flexibility in the ART regimen in the composition of the NRTI base pair in the 3-drug, 2-drug class options. Guidelines by the IAS-USA differ in that it recommends 3 options for initial therapy. Within the recommendations, 2 of the options use tenofovir alafenamide (TAF)-based NRTI pairing versus tenofovir disoproxil (TDF)-based NRTI pairing offered in the DHHS guidelines. Although virologically similar, this recommendation was made based on evidence that the lower plasma levels and higher intracellular concentration of the tenofovir component result in fewer renal and bone toxic effects compared with TDF.[19] In the event that first-line regimens are not available or not an option, both organizations provide recommendations on alternative regimens that may be used to select a regimen that is optimal for viral suppression based on an individual's circumstances.

It currently is recommended that all individuals diagnosed with HIV be started on ART immediately to increase adherence, reduce associated morbidity and mortality, prevent future transmissions, and accelerate ART-mediated viral suppression.[16,17] ART initiation should not be delayed, especially in individuals with AIDS-defining conditions, who are pregnant, or with acute or recent HIV infection.[16,17] If the individual is ready, ART should be initiated anywhere between the day of diagnosis to the first days after being diagnosed.[16,17] The initiation of ART should be delayed only if there are significant barriers to adherence or the presence of comorbidities that prohibit ART.

Guidelines for Treatment in Pregnancy

All women who are pregnant and HIV positive should be treated with ART despite CD4 cell count or viral load to maintain viral suppression throughout pregnancy and prevent perinatal transmission. The recommendations differ based on whether a woman is pregnant and has never received ART versus a woman already taking ART (**Box 3**).[16,17,20] Women who become pregnant who already have an ART regimen

---

Box 3
First-line antiretroviral therapy recommendations during pregnancy

Initial regimen in pregnancy
- Dolutegravir/abacavir/lamivudine
- Dolutegravir + TDF/emtricitabine or TDF/lamivudine
- Raltegravir + (abacavir/lamivudine or TDF/emtricitabine or tenofovir disoproxmil/lamivudine)
- Atazanavir/ritonavir + (abacavir/lamivudine or TDF/emtricitabine or TDF/lamivudine)
- Darunavir/ritonavir + (abacavir/lamivudine or TDF/emtricitabine or TDF/lamivudine)

Pregnancy in the presence of an established, suppressive regimen
- ART regimen changes should be considered for regimens containing due to insufficient data:
  ○ Bictegravir
  ○ Doravirine
  ○ Ibalizumab
  ○ Bictegravir/emtricitabine/TAF
  ○ Doravirine/lamivudine/TDF
- Consider switching or frequently monitor HIV RNA for ART regimens containing:
  ○ Boosted elvitegravir
  ○ Atazanavir boosted by cobicistat
  ○ Darunavir boosted by cobicistat
- All other regimens may be continued.

---

should have their regimen evaluated to ensure that it is appropriate for pregnancy.[17,20] One of the most recent concerns was related to the development of neural tube defects in the presence of dolutegravir. This concern was based on preliminary findings that suggested that there was an increased risk of neural tube defects in infants born to women on dolutegravir-containing regimens. The 2019 DHHS updated guidelines continue to include dolutegravir in preferred regimens for pregnant women because subsequent findings reported a prevalence of neural tube defects.[16,20] It is recommended, however, that all women of childbearing age are advised of this potential adverse effect as the prevalence continues to be higher than women who are on non–dolutegravir-containing regimens.[16,20] The IAS-USA supports the World Health Organization recommendation that women of childbearing age who wish to become pregnant or do not have a reliable contraceptive method should avoid dolutegravir.[17,21]

Guidelines for Treatment of Children

Treatment-naïve infants and children less than 12 years of age should receive an ART regimen that includes an NRTI base pair and either an NNRTI, INSTI, or boosted PI.[22] The NRTI base pair selected is based on the age of the child. It consists of either zidovudine or TDF plus either emtricitabine or lamivudine.[22]

- For infants less than 14 days old, the recommended regimen is an NRTI base pair and nevirapine.
- For children between 14 days and 3 years old, the recommended regimen is an NRTI base pair plus lopinavir boosted with ritonavir. If a child weighs more than 2 kg, raltegravir may be used instead.
- For children between 3 years and 12 years old, the recommended regimen is an NRTI base pair plus an additional drug based on weight. For those weighing less than 25 kg, boosted atazanavir or twice-daily boosted darunavir is an option. For those weighing more than 25 kg, either dolutegravir or elvitegravir boosted with cobicistat is an option.[22]

Just as with adults, children may have circumstances that prevent them from accessing or being able to use first-line regimens to treat HIV. For these situations, the DHHS has provided alternative regimens that are just as effective in the viral suppression of HIV.[22]

LABORATORY MONITORING

Baseline laboratory testing should be performed on entry to HIV care and prior to ART initiation. These tests include, but are not limited to, a comprehensive metabolic panel, complete blood cell count, hepatic serologies, sexually transmitted infection screening, urinalysis, HIV-1 RNA, and CD4 cell count and percentage.[16–18] This testing provides the health care provider with the necessary information to gauge adherence as well as monitor any adverse effects that may be attributed to ART. Genotypic resistance testing also should be ordered to assist the provider in the selection of an appropriate ART regimen that is best suited to suppress that person's virus.[18,19] After baseline results are acquired, subsequent and ongoing laboratory testing should be performed as clinically indicated (**Table 3**).[16,17] Assessment of viral suppression and immune function can monitored with 2 laboratory tests, specifically, HIV-1 RNA and CD4 cell count and percentage, respectively. The goal of viral suppression depends on the recommending body. The IAS-USA notes that an HIV RNA less than 50 copies/mL is achievement of viral suppression compared with the DHHS who uses the goal of less than 200 copies/mL.[16,17] The threshold of less than 200 copies/mL is supported by guidelines from the AIDS Clinical Trials Group that states that this threshold eliminates most cases of viremia.[16,23] An HIV RNA at either of these goals is sufficient, especially if suppression is maintained for more than a year. The CD4 cell count and percentage initially assist the health care provider with determining if there is a need for prophylaxis against opportunistic infections. Once viral suppression is acquired for more than 1 year to 2 years, CD4 cell count and percentage are optional.[16,17]

Table 3 Laboratory monitoring	
Laboratory Test	**Frequency**
HLA-B*5701	Baseline only
CD4 cell count and percentage[a] HIV RNA level	1. Baseline 2. Six wk after the initiation of ART or a new regimen 3. Every 3 mo until viral suppression, then every 6 mo
Gonorrhea Chlamydia Syphilis Hepatitis serologies	1. Baseline 2. At least annually for all sexually active patients More frequent screening (every 3–6 mo) for persons at higher risk
Hemoglobin A$_{1c}$ Comprehensive metabolic panel Complete blood cell count	1. Baseline 2. Within 3 mo of starting new ART regimen 3. Annually
Urinalysis	1. Baseline 2. Annually
HIV genotypic resistance testing Viral tropism	Virologic failure, as applicable

[a] Once CD4 cell count is >250 cells/μL and viral suppression achieved for 1 y, monitoring becomes optional as long as viral suppression continues.

Viral suppression typically can be achieved in a maximum of 6 months. There are instances, however, where this is not the case and there presents a concern of virologic failure. With the technological advancements in the formulation of newer ART regimens, virologic failure is becoming less common. It is possible, however, for it to occur due to genotypic mutations, drug-drug interactions, ART modification secondary to drug toxicities, and issues related to adherence.[16,17] In these instances, it is necessary for a holistic review of potential barriers along with genotypic resistance testing to determine if an alternative regimen needs to be selected.

SUPPORTIVE CARE

For health care providers, it is imperative that they provide supportive care to PLWH. This includes addressing related issues that traditionally may not be covered. These issues include, but are not limited to, mental health, substance abuse, cost, and correctional care. Mental health is essential to the success of self-care of a PLWH. Unmanaged mental illness can serve as a major barrier to adherence of any plan related to HIV. Substance abuse can hasten disease progression and affect ART adherence, with the potential to exacerbate complications related to HIV. Health care providers must encourage adherence to all therapy or rehabilitation, nonpharmacologic or pharmacologic, to assist in a person's ability to adhere to ART and achieve viral suppression. PLWH experience an increased amount of stigma, discrimination, and shame that contribute to their overall mental health. There may be a lack in social support systems related to this stigma, which have a further negative impact on mental health. This presents as being treated differently by family, friends, colleagues, and health care providers. It is essential that health care providers and staff provide health care environments that ensure confidentiality, emotional support, and cultural sensitivity and humility. Additionally, providing support in the form of resources (eg, peer educators or nonmedical support organizations) to assist with health care navigation and the lived experience of living with HIV increase rapport.

One major challenge with HIV management and ART adherence is cost of care. Whether insured, underinsured, or uninsured, there are direct and indirect costs associated with managing HIV. The most direct and relevant direct cost is accessibility to ART. There can be issues with access to what insurance carriers are willing to cover based on similar virologic efficacy versus a health care provider's desire for a safer adverse-effect profile.[19] Another direct cost to consider is the cost of medical visits because visit frequency is determined by adherence, immune function, and the need for additional monitoring. Indirect costs to consider include but are not limited to the cost of transportation, work absences for appointments, and accessibility of specialists for HIV-related complications.

Lastly, health care providers must consider how to provide care in less traditional settings, such as custodial care. PLWH who may need to serve time in custodial care for a period of time continue to need access to ART. Health care providers should work diligently to reduce any barriers related to the transition into custodial care, during the period of incarceration, and exiting custodial care. It The types of barriers to be addressed also depend on the type of correctional care a patient is entering—jail or prison. Jail typically involves a sentence of less than a year. Prison typically involves a sentence longer than a year. The prison setting lends to an increased chance in continuity of care compared with that of a jail setting due to the length of stay in the custodial facility.

SUMMARY

Knowledge of the pathophysiology of HIV and risk factors that lead to its acquisition is vital to the health care provider's ability to provide holistic care to PLWH as well as those at risk. Such holistic care also is impacted by a provider's understanding of individual characteristics, social norms, and structural barriers that serve as barriers to preventive efforts. Implementing the treatment as prevention strategy is important because it promotes viral suppression among PLWH and reduces the likelihood of HIV acquisition among those at highest risk. Attacking such barriers with this understanding, coupled with the continuous evolvement of pharmacologic regimens, is key to reducing HIV incidence in the future and ending the epidemic.

DISCLOSURE

The authors have nothing to disclose.

REFERENCES

1. Centers for Disease Control and Prevention. HIV in the United States and dependent areas. 2019. Available at: https://www.cdc.gov/hiv/statistics/overview/ataglance.html. Accessed December 30, 2019.
2. Centers for Disease Control and Prevention. HIV Surveillance report, 2016; 28. 2017. Available at: http://www.cdc.gov/hiv/library/reports/hiv-surveillance.html. Accessed December 30, 2019.
3. United States Department of Health and Human Services. AIDSinfo glossary of HIV/AIDS-related terms. 9th edition. 2018. Available at: https://aidsinfo.nih.gov/contentfiles/glossaryhivrelatedterms_english.pdf. Accessed December 30, 2019.
4. Centers for Disease Control and Prevention. About HIV/AIDS. 2019. Available at: https://www.cdc.gov/hiv/basics/whatishiv.html. Accessed December 30, 2019.
5. AIDSinfo. The stages of HIV infection. 2019. Available at: https://aidsinfo.nih.gov/understanding-hiv-aids/fact-sheets/19/46/the-stages-of-hiv-infection. Accessed December 30, 2019.
6. Centers for Disease Control and Prevention. Revised surveillance case definition for HIV infection – United States, 2014. MMWR Recomm Rep 2014;63(RR03):1–10. Available at: https://www.cdc.gov/mmwr/preview/mmwrhtml/rr6303a1.htm. Accessed December 30, 2019.
7. Centers for Disease Control and Prevention. Revised surveillance case definitions for HIV infection among adults, adolescents, and children aged <18 months and for HIV infection and AIDS among children aged 18 months to <13 years – United States, 2008. MMWR Recomm Rep 2008;57(RR10):1–8. Available at: https://www.cdc.gov/mmwr/preview/mmwrhtml/rr5710a1.htm. Accessed December 30, 2019.
8. AIDSinfo. HIV/AIDS: The basics. 2019. Available at: https://aidsinfo.nih.gov/understanding-hiv-aids/fact-sheets/19/45/hiv-aids–the-basics. Accessed December 30, 2019.
9. World Health Organization. HIV/AIDS. 2019. Available at: https://www.who.int/news-room/fact-sheets/detail/hiv-aids. Accessed December 30, 2019.
10. Hargreaves J, Delany-Moretlwe S, Hallett TB, et al. The HIV prevention cascade: integrating theories of epidemiological, behavioral, and social science into programme design and monitoring. Lancet HIV 2016;7(3):e318–22.
11. Pantelic M, Stegling C, Shackleton S, et al. Power to participants: a call for person-centred HIV prevention services and research. J Int AIDS Soc 2018; 21(S7):e25167.
12. Landovitz R, Currier J. Postexposure Prophylaxis for HIV infection. N Engl J Med 2009;361:1768–75.

13. Centers for Disease Control and Prevention. PEP 101. 2019. Available at: https://www.cdc.gov/hiv/basics/pep.html. Accessed December 31, 2019.
14. Desia M, Field N, Grant R, et al. Recent advances in pre-exposure prophylaxis for HIV. BMJ 2017;359:j5011.
15. Centers for Disease Control and Prevention. Understanding the Continuum of Care. 2019. Available at: https://www.cdc.gov/hiv/pdf/library/factsheets/cdc-hiv-care-continuum.pdf. Accessed December 31, 2019.
16. Panel on antiretroviral guidelines for adults and adolescents. Guidelines for the use of antiretroviral agents in adults and adolescents with HIV. Department of Health and Human Services; 2019. Available at: http://www.aidsinfo.nih.gov/ContentFiles/AdultandAdolescentGL.pdf. Accessed January 1, 2020.
17. Saag M, Benson C, Gandhi R, et al. Antiretroviral Drugs for Treatment and Prevention of HIV Infection in Adults 2018 Recommendations of the International Antiviral Society–USA Panel. JAMA 2018;320(4):379–96.
18. Pitts C. Updates on the pharmacologic treatment of individuals with human immunodeficiency virus. Nurs Clin North Am 2016;51:45–56.
19. Sax PE, Pozniak A, Montes ML, et al. Coformulated bictegravir, emtricitabine, and tenofovir alafenamide versus dolutegravir with emtricitabine and tenofovir alafenamide, for initial treatment of HIV-1 infection (GS-US-380-1490): a randomised, double-blind, multicentre, phase 3, non-inferiority trial. Lancet 2017;390(10107): 2073–82.
20. Panel on treatment of pregnant women with HIV infection and prevention of perinatal transmission. Recommendations for use of antiretroviral drugs in transmission in the United States. 2019. Available at: http://aidsinfo.nih.gov/contentfiles/lvguidelines/PerinatalGL.pdf. Accessed January 1, 2020.
21. World Health Organization (WHO). Potential safety issue affecting women living with HIV using dolutegravir at the time of conception. 2018. Available at: http://www.who.int/medicines/publications/drugalerts/Statement_on_DTG _18May_ 2018final.pdf. Accessed July 4, 2018.
22. Panel on antiretroviral therapy and medical management of children living with HIV. Guidelines for the use of antiretroviral agents in pediatric HIV infection. 2019. Available at: http://aidsinfo.nih.gov/contentfiles/lvguidelines/pediatricguidelines.pdf. Accessed January 1, 2020.
23. Ribaudo H, Lennox J, Currier J, et al. Virologic failure endpoint definition in clinical trials: Is using HIV-1 RNA threshold <200 copies/mL better than <50 copies/mL? An analysis of ACTG studies. 16th Conference on Retroviruses and Opportunistic Infections. Montreal, Canada, February 8–11, 2009.

Pharmacoprevention of Human Immunodeficiency Virus Infection

Charles Yingling, DNP, FNP-BC[a],*, Cindy Broholm, MS, MPH, FNP-BC[b],
Shirley Stephenson, MS, MFA, MA, FNP-BC[c]

KEYWORDS

- PrEP • nPEP • PEP • HIV prevention • Pharmacoprevention

KEY POINTS

- Human immunodeficiency virus (HIV) preexposure prophylaxis (PrEP) is the most effective way to prevent new HIV infections.
- HIV nonoccupational postexposure prophylaxis (nPEP) is an important strategy for preventing HIV in people who have been exposed.
- Nurses of all levels have a role in offering both HIV PrEP and nPEP.

INTRODUCTION

Modern pharmacoprevention for infectious diseases (ie, the use of pharmaceuticals to prevent infection with a pathogen) dates back to the early use of quinine for malaria prophylaxis in the seventeenth century.[1] Since that time, pharmacoprevention has expanded to address numerous infectious diseases, including influenza, varicella, and hepatitis B. Pharmacoprevention of human immunodeficiency virus (HIV) has gained attention in recent years because, absent a vaccine, this is currently the most efficacious approach to prevent new HIV infections globally.

Work on pharmacoprevention of HIV began in the mid-1990s and focused on the prevention of mother-to-child transmission (PMTCT)[2] and prevention of health care workers contracting HIV from accidental percutaneous exposures.[3] Clinical guidelines for the use of medications for occupational HIV infection were available as early as 1998[4] and PMTCT guidelines followed in 2004.[5] With growing evidence for the efficacy

[a] Department of Population Health Nursing Science, University of Illinois at Chicago College of Nursing, 845 South Damen Avenue, Chicago, IL 60612, USA; [b] Harriet Rothkopf Heilbrunn School of Nursing, Long Island University, 1 University Plaza, Brooklyn, NY 11201, USA; [c] Department of Population Health Nursing Science, University of Illinois at Chicago College of Nursing, 3240 West Division Street, Chicago, IL 60651, USA
* Corresponding author.
E-mail address: cyingl1@uic.edu
Twitter: @CharlieUIC (C.Y.)

Nurs Clin N Am 55 (2020) 429–444
https://doi.org/10.1016/j.cnur.2020.06.006
0029-6465/20/© 2020 Elsevier Inc. All rights reserved.
nursing.theclinics.com

of HIV pharmacoprevention in newborns and health care workers, the focus of research in this area shifted to identifying an effective strategy to prevent new HIV infections in those who may be exposed outside of a health care setting.[6] This most recent stage of HIV prevention work has identified 3 strategies for the pharmacoprevention of nonoccupationally acquired HIV: treatment as prevention (TasP), preexposure prophylaxis (PrEP), and nonoccupational postexposure prophylaxis (nPEP). TasP is based on the evidence that the risk of HIV transmission from an individual with HIV who has an undetectable viral load is effectively zero.[7–10] This concept of undetectable equals untransmittable is known as U = U. Because TasP involves treatment of HIV, this article focuses on PrEP and nPEP, interventions that nurses can offer in a wide range of settings.

PURPOSE

Using a case-based approach, this article describes the epidemiology and population disparities in HIV incidence, presents current evidence surrounding the efficacy of PrEP and nPEP, provides an overview of risk assessment and prescribing so that nurses of all levels can confidently participate in and adopt these effective interventions in their practice, and reviews best practices in treatment retention for people at high risk of HIV.

EPIDEMIOLOGY AND DISPARITIES

The Centers for Disease Control and Prevention (CDC) estimates that, in the United States, there were 1,140,400 adults and adolescents living with HIV and 38,739 new HIV infections in 2017.[11] Although the overall incidence of new HIV infections in the United States remained stable between 2012 and 2016, it is important to look more closely at the populations affected by HIV to understand trends and populations that can benefit from targeted prevention efforts. There are 4 primary groups that are disproportionately infected with HIV: men who have sex with men (MSM), people of color (particularly black and Latinx), transgender women (ie, individuals with male sex assigned at birth who identify as women), and people who live in the southern portion of the United States.

Intersectionality amplifies risk in these populations. For example, a transgender woman of color who resides in the South would have a much higher risk of HIV infection than a white MSM living in the Midwest. Structural racism, systems that perpetuate racial inequities, further contributes to these disparities because communities of color are less likely to have access to health insurance and primary health care services (**Box 1**).[12]

Box 1
Clinical case, part 1

Clinical case

Noah is a 29-year-old man who presents to your practice requesting PrEP. He identifies as bisexual, and is currently in a relationship with Meredith, who tends bar at the restaurant where he is a chef. Occasionally Noah and Meredith invite Trevor, a man with whom they work, to join them for sex. Neither man wears condoms when having intercourse with one another, or with Meredith, who uses an intrauterine device for contraception. Trevor has told them that he has other female and male partners, and rarely uses condoms.

EFFICACY OF PREEXPOSURE PROPHYLAXIS AND NONOCCUPATIONAL POSTEXPOSURE PROPHYLAXIS

A significant body of evidence supports the efficacy of HIV PrEP and nPEP. Given accumulated data, the CDC now asserts that HIV PrEP is 99% effective at preventing HIV infection from sexual exposure when taken daily[13]. This effectiveness rate is derived from several foundational studies and real-world experience since the first PrEP treatment was approved in 2012.[14] If started within 72 hours of exposure, nPEP is very effective.[15–17] Because of ethical concerns regarding withholding treatment from people who have been exposed to HIV, evidence for nPEP is based on observational studies and animal models. So, although nPEP is highly effective, it is difficult to quantify its efficacy.[15]

Given the evidence that attests to the efficacy of PrEP and nPEP for the prevention of HIV, global consensus supports that these 2 pharmacoprevention strategies should be part of routine clinical practice.[14,18] In 2019, the US Preventive Services Task Force (USPSTF) released a grade A recommendation for the use of PrEP for the prevention of HIV.[19] Postexposure prophylaxis guidelines were first released by the CDC in 2005 and updated in 2016. The World Health Organization (WHO) nPEP guidelines were first released in 2006 and updated in 2014 (**Box 2**).

STRATEGIES TO PROMOTE EFFICIENT UPTAKE OF HUMAN IMMUNODEFICIENCY VIRUS PHARMACOPREVENTION
Preexposure Prophylaxis

In 2012, the US Food and Drug Administration approved a single combination pill for HIV PrEP: tenofovir disoproxil fumarate/emtricitabine (TDF/FTC) taken daily to prevent HIV infection. In 2019, 1 additional product, tenofovir alafenamide/emtricitabine (TAF/FTC), was approved for HIV PrEP for sexual exposure excluding receptive vaginal sex.[20] Despite PrEP providing an estimated efficacy of almost 99% in preventing HIV infection, the overall rates of new HIV infections did not decline between 2012 and 2016,[13,21] likely because people who would benefit from PrEP are not receiving it. In 2015, approximately 1.1 million people in the United States would have benefitted from PrEP. However, only about 90,000 prescriptions for PrEP were filled that year.[22] In addition, there are significant disparities in who is receiving this important prevention tool. It was estimated that, during the study period, approximately 44% of the people who could have potentially benefitted from PrEP were African American, but

---

Box 2
Clinical case, part 2

In your clinic, Noah explains that it is difficult for him to get away from the restaurant, and he would like to receive his prescription for PrEP today. He reports a negative rapid HIV test about 2 months ago. His past medical history includes syphilis, which was treated with 3 doses of benzathine penicillin G. Noah has no allergies, and his only medication is 600 mg of ibuprofen, taken every few days for back pain. He drinks 2 cups of coffee each morning and a half a bottle of wine most nights, after the restaurant closes. He and Meredith smoke marijuana 3 times per week. He has never used other recreational drugs, tobacco, or electronic cigarettes. Noah considers himself to be in good health except for fatigue and muscle aches, which he attributes to working long hours on his feet in a high-stress environment. He denies a history of kidney disease; hepatitis B infection; or recent rash, fever, and malaise. His last condomless, receptive anal intercourse was with Trevor approximately 4 weeks ago. Noah is concerned about how often he will need to return for appointments.

only 1% of them received a prescription, and of Latinx people, only 3% of those who might have benefitted were prescribed PrEP.[22] This finding indicates the need to increase the uptake of PrEP in the United States and to address disparities in access among vulnerable populations. Nurses of all levels, as the largest and most trusted health profession in the United States, can play an important role in promoting HIV pharmacoprevention. Increasing awareness and confidence among nurses may help turn the tide of inequity in PrEP prescribing and other risk reduction efforts.

Although communities at high risk need concerted outreach and access to HIV prevention services, all patients need to be assessed and offered methods to reduce HIV risk. Assessment for risk of HIV infection requires inquiry about sexual behaviors and drug use, two topics that patients and nurses may be uncomfortable discussing. The patient interview to assess HIV risk must include questions about injection drug use, partners with whom the patient has sex (men, women, or both), whether the individual has multiple partners, and whether the patient's partners have other partners. Helpful tools that provide guidance on assessing HIV risk are the GOALS framework for taking a sexual history in primary care,[23] CDC's *A Guide to Taking a Sexual History*,[24] and the Assessing Risk for Contracting HIV (ARCH-IDU) Risk Scoring Sheet.[25]

It is critical that clinicians know that PrEP is appropriate for anyone who states they are at risk of acquiring HIV, even if they do not disclose specifics about the potential for exposure, and for anyone who anticipates risk in the near future.[26] In a discussion of PrEP suitability in primary care settings, O'Byrne[27] recommended 2 simple considerations: is there a chance of HIV exposure, and, if so, would that individual's practices enable HIV transmission? Steps that may facilitate comfort and patient-provider rapport include a patient-centered approach; practitioner openness; shared decision making; stigma-free language; opportunities for new patients to nonverbally disclose information; and clinic displays that address HIV, sexual orientation, gender affirmation, sexually transmitted infections (STIs), substance use, and other sensitive topics.[28,29]

Risk compensation

Nurses and other health care professionals may be concerned that the protection conferred by PrEP will increase risk behaviors such as condomless sex or needle sharing (ie, risk compensation).[30] Some studies have shown an increase in sexual risk compensation among people who use PrEP.[31] However, similar to the way in which providers do not withhold oral contraceptives from women for fear of decreased condom use, a concern for risk compensation should never be used as a reason to not offer PrEP. Instead, engagement in care while receiving PrEP may ultimately result in a decrease in both HIV and other STI transmission, because of routine testing and early treatment of asymptomatic infections.[32]

Current approved agents and regimens

TDF/FTC is approved for prevention of HIV in people aged 13 years and older who weigh at least 35 kg and who have risk of exposure via sexual or injection drug use. In 2019, TAF/FTC was approved for prevention of HIV via sexual exposure excluding receptive vaginal sex and intravenous drug use.[33] Because there are no data for the use of TAF/FTC in receptive vaginal sex or injection drug use, at this point, TAF/FTC should not be prescribed for HIV prevention in these populations.

In 2019, the WHO released guidance for the use of TDF/FTC-based event-driven PrEP for MSM.[34] Instead of daily dosing, event-driven PrEP is only taken when a possible HIV exposure may occur. Event-driven PrEP is also called a 2 + 1 + 1 regimen (ie, 2 tablets taken between 2 and 24 hours before the possible exposure, then 1 tablet 24 hours later, and another 48 hours later). If additional exposures occur, TDF/FTC is continued daily until 48 hours after the last exposure.[34,35] In MSM, this approach was found to be 97% to 100% effective in reducing HIV incidence.[36] The dosing regimen has not been sufficiently studied in other populations (eg, heterosexual women, transgender women, and people who inject drugs). Thus, it is only recommended in MSM.[26,35] It is also important to note that event-driven PrEP is currently off label in both the United States and Canada.

Several other options for PrEP are under investigation, including oral formulations, long-acting injectables, and microbicide rings and gels. However, none are expected to be available until at least 2021.[37]

Time to protection
A common patient concern is how long it takes for PrEP to be effective. Time to protection data are based on pharmacokinetic modeling, not on clinical outcome studies. Therefore, a conclusive interval is not known. Clinical outcome studies[36] have informed guidance, particularly around the use of a loading dose to decrease time to protection for rectal exposures. The CDC recommends 7 days for rectal exposure and 20 days for vaginal and blood exposure.[14] However, based on more recent modeling data, the 2017 WHO and 2018 British HIV Association guidelines recommend that protection is afforded after 7 days for both blood and vaginal exposure as well as rectal exposure.[38] Nurses should refer to the most recent data and counsel patients about what is and is not known so that patients can make informed decisions.

Prescribing/dispensing preexposure prophylaxis
Nurses of all levels can provide access to PrEP. Advanced practice registered nurses can prescribe the regimen and registered nurses (RNs) can order the regimen using standing order sets.[39] The WHO and Canadian and United States health authorities all have issued comprehensive prescribing guidelines for PrEP regimens and these should serve as nurses' primary source for PrEP prescribing/dispensing.[14,40,41]

The first steps in identifying people who will benefit from PrEP are risk assessment and screening for contraindications. However, as stated earlier, any individual who seeks PrEP should be provided with a prescription if there are no contraindications. HIV infection is an absolute contraindication to PrEP. Assuming a person is HIV negative, a contraindication for the initiation of FTC/TDF-based PrEP is a creatinine clearance (CrCl) less than 60 mL/min. Because of its favorable renal safety profile, FTC/TAF-based PrEP can be initiated in MSM and transgender women with a CrCl greater than 30 mL/min.[42] All current medications should be reviewed to assess for any interactions, particularly with nephrotoxic agents.[14,40,41]

Initial assessment for PrEP should include any high-risk encounters that occurred in the last 4 weeks, symptoms of acute HIV infection (ie, fever, night sweats, lymphadenopathy, rash, diarrhea) in the last 6 weeks, as well as hepatitis B virus (HBV) and pregnancy status. For individuals with a high-risk encounter in the last 72 hours, nPEP should be given for a month before PrEP. For a person with a high-risk encounter in the past 4 weeks or symptoms suggestive of acute HIV infection, an HIV viral load is indicated to rule out HIV infection.

HBV infection is not a contraindication to PrEP. However, the 2 current medications for PrEP are also treatments for HBV. Therefore, education on the risk of rebound viremia and the need for continued HBV treatment at the time of PrEP discontinuation is critical. Women at risk of HIV infection who are pregnant, considering pregnancy, or breastfeeding may take PrEP, but the nurse and patient should discuss risks and benefits. The rates of birth defects in women on TDF/FTC are not increased compared with the general population.[43] In addition, the WHO provides clear guidance that breastfeeding while taking TDF/FTC is appropriate.[44]

Certain social factors may make some providers reluctant to prescribe PrEP. Although substance use, inconsistent condom use, mental illness, intimate partner violence, insecure housing, and other factors may present additional challenges for adherence, they are not reasons to decline a PrEP prescription.[26] Appropriate support services and/or referrals should be provided to optimize success for all individuals.

There are 2 approaches to starting PrEP: rapid start (ie, same-day) and conventional start. A patient is a candidate for a rapid start if they have no symptoms of acute HIV infection and initial laboratory specimens (**Table 1**) have been collected with results available within 1 week. An individual with a high-risk exposure within the past 72 hours

---

Table 1
Initial laboratory tests for preexposure prophylaxis and nonoccupational postexposure prophylaxis

PrEP	PEP	Comments
Baseline HIV test	Baseline HIV test	• Fourth-generation HIV (third-generation alternative) • Point-of-care rapid HIV (recommended if available for rapid start of PrEP) Retest 1 mo after initiation (PrEP) if high-risk encounter in past 4 wk Retest every 3 mo (PrEP)
HIV NAT (viral load)	HIV NAT (viral load)	If high-risk exposure in past 4 wk or symptoms of acute HIV in past 6 wk
Serum creatinine and calculated (CrCl)	—	TDF/FTC contraindicated if CrCl <60 mL/min TAF/FTC contraindicated if CrCl <30 mL/min Retest every 6 mo
HBsAg, anti-HBs, anti-HBc-IgG, HAV	HBsAg, anti-HBs, anti-HBc-IgG	Vaccinate nonimmune Chronic HBV: consider referral to HBV specialist
HCV serology	—	Chronic hepatitis C: refer for treatment
STI testing (syphilis, GC, CT)	STI testing (syphilis, GC, CT)	Initially Retest every 3 mo (PrEP) unless low risk For MSM and transgender women, routinely perform 3-site testing for GC/CT (rectal, oral, genital)
Pregnancy test (all individuals of childbearing capacity)	Pregnancy test (all individuals of childbearing capacity)	Discuss importance of preventing HIV during pregnancy and risks/benefits of PrEP or PEP. TDF/FTC not shown to increase risk of birth defects
UA Liver enzymes	—	Optional

For most patients, the authors recommend doing the laboratory tests necessary for PrEP when prescribing PEP so that they can be transitioned to PrEP after a month of PEP.

Abbreviations: Anti-HBs, hepatitis B surface antibody; anti-HBc, hepatitis B core antibody; anti-HBC, hepatitis C antibody; CT, chlamydia trachomatis; GC, neisseria gonorrhoeae; HAV, hepatitis A virus IgM; HBsAg, hepatitis B surface antigen; HCV, hepatitis C virus; IgG, immunoglobulin G; NAT, nucleic acid test; UA, urinalysis.

Data from Centers for Disease Control and Prevention. Preexposure Prophylaxis for the Prevention of HIV Infection in the United States - 2017 Update: A Clinical Practice Guideline. Atlanta; 2017. And WHO. Consolidated Guidelines on the Use of Antiretroviral Drugs for Treating and Preventing HIV Infection. http://apps.who.int/iris/bitstream/10665/85322/1/WHO_HIV_2013.7_eng.pdf. Published 2016. Accessed January 2, 2020.

should receive nPEP instead of PrEP for a month to prevent infection and then transition to PrEP if clinically appropriate. For people with symptoms of possible acute HIV infection, known renal disease, or a history of HBV, initiation of PrEP should be delayed until laboratory results are received. As with contraception, delayed initiation of PrEP results in missed prevention opportunities and the possibility of patients becoming lost to follow-up.[45,46] So, whenever possible, the nurse should offer rapid-start PrEP to eligible patients. If an individual who received a rapid-start prescription tests positive for HIV, the regimen should be intensified for complete HIV treatment as soon as possible.

Selection of PrEP regimen should be guided by patient risk factors and exposure sites. TDF/FTC is the most appropriate choice for most people seeking PrEP. TAF/FTC may be an option for MSM and transgender women, particularly in the context of impaired renal function. An important resource to assist in navigating complex clinical situations for PrEP initiation or management is the CDC PrEPLine (855-HIV-PrEP). This free service provides expert guidance for clinicians who are prescribing/dispensing PrEP (**Box 3**).

Box 3
Clinical case, part 3

Based on Noah's reported history, his access to a reliable phone, and your ability to receive laboratory results within 3 days, you provided a same-day prescription for PrEP. You counseled Noah that he would not be protected until he had taken TDF/FTC daily for 1 week and that, if he were to have a positive HIV test, you would need to change his regimen and obtain additional blood tests. Noah expressed an understanding and agreed to this plan. He also stated an interest in bringing his partner Meredith to a future appointment, to see whether she might consider PrEP.

Preexposure prophylaxis patient education Patient education should address potential side effects, including the possibility of renal impairment and a reversible decrease in bone density with TDF/FTC. Although no associated fractures have been documented, this may be a consideration for older individuals, for those with a history of osteoporosis, and adolescents that have not reached the age of bone maturation. Anticipatory guidance regarding common initial medication side effects, such as nausea, flatulence, and headache, should be given. Most people tolerate PrEP well and do not experience a so-called startup syndrome. For those who do, side effects typically resolve within 3 months and can be treated symptomatically.[47] Key points for patients considering PrEP are that less-than-daily dosing may diminish protection, and continued PrEP use after becoming infected with HIV may contribute to drug resistance. Counseling should also focus on other forms of risk reduction, including condoms. As with nonbarrier forms of contraception, PrEP does not prevent other STIs. Clinicians should counsel patients to take a missed pill as soon as it is remembered, unless it is time for the next dose, in which case it should be skipped. Although 100% adherence is the goal, an occasional missed dose should be normalized.[14] For MSM preferring event-based PrEP dosing, the nurse should counsel that this is an off-label use of the medication.

Preexposure prophylaxis in the context of hormone therapy For individuals using feminizing hormones for gender affirmation, it is important to counsel on the greater importance of PrEP adherence. Concurrent dosing of exogenous estrogen and TDF/FTC can reduce serum levels of TDF. This reduction is not clinically significant in terms of reduced protection, but it is significant in that there is less forgiveness for missed doses. In our clinical practice caring for transgender women, some patients have expressed concerns based on hearsay that TDF/FTC reduce levels of estrogen. This hearsay is not accurate, and reassurance can be provided to transgender women on feminizing hormones who desire PrEP.[48]

Access and adherence to preexposure prophylaxis PrEP is 1 element of a comprehensive, patient-centered, personalized program of HIV prevention. An understanding of the individual's overall well-being and motivations better enables the practitioner and care team to assess readiness, and support adherence.[26,49,50] Some considerations include the patient's understanding of HIV, reasons for wanting PrEP, support network, housing and food security, medication history and past adherence patterns, availability of a safe place to keep medication, risk of intimate partner violence, and possible consequences if someone finds the medication. Challenges in any of these areas are not reasons to delay prophylaxis. Appropriate support and/or referrals should be given, including linkage to payment assistance programs. The retail cost of TDF/FTC without insurance ranges from $1500 to $2000/mo. Of note, the lifetime treatment cost of HIV infection is estimated to be $379,668.[51] Many states and localities have programs to support PrEP access. In the United States, the Department of Health and Human Services offers PrEP at no cost to people without insurance (https://www.getyourprep.com/).

Follow-up care All individuals using PrEP should have follow-up, either in person or virtually within 30 days after initiation and laboratory tests every 3 months thereafter. The 30-day follow-up is an opportunity to assess adherence and evaluate renal function in those at risk for impairment (ie, people with diabetes, chronic kidney disease, hypertension, or age>65 years). A repeat HIV test is also indicated at this time. Subsequent encounters should include repeat HIV testing, including viral load testing if there are symptoms of acute HIV infection. In addition, these encounters are opportunities for STI screening based on client sexual practices. Multisite STI testing should be performed according to locations of sexual activity (eg, oral, genital, anal). However, given the high rates of extragenital STIs (ie, oral and rectal) among MSM and transgender women, the authors recommend routine testing of all sites.[40] Self-collected rectal and vaginal swabs have comparable accuracy with clinician-collected swabs.[52,53] Pregnancy testing should be considered in cisgender women and any individual who may become pregnant. Renal function should be evaluated every 6 months. For those at risk for hepatitis C virus (HCV) infection, annual HCV screening is indicated.

Various factors may influence visit intervals. Ideally, visit scheduling is a joint decision by both the nurse and patient. Adolescents and individuals with adherence challenges should have more frequent contact for supportive counseling. However, these same patients often face the most barriers to attending appointments. Communication via phone, telehealth, or an electronic health record portal can be useful to supplement in-person visits. A collaborative care approach that includes behavioral health, peer support groups, and case management services optimizes face-to-face clinic visits. Combining PrEP visits with routine health maintenance, such as immunizations, and women's health, also streamlines care. PrEP education and provision naturally dovetail with family planning visits, which should address STI prevention. As with contraception, PrEP can both empower women and reduce risk.[54]

Quarterly HIV and STI screening and biannual creatinine clearance are recommended for all patients on PrEP. However, a face-to-face encounter may not be necessary for patients who report excellent adherence, no side effects and have stable personal circumstances. However, it is important to communicate often enough to assess risk, and address new patient concerns. For example, someone in a long-term relationship who is adherent with PrEP may develop concerns about their partner's fidelity and desire more frequent STI testing, whereas someone with a seropositive partner may decide to discontinue PrEP because the partner's HIV viral load has been consistently undetectable. Understanding U = U enables practitioners to appropriately counsel patients on risk. Likewise, U = U offers patients another crucial reason to encourage treatment adherence for their partners with HIV (**Box 4**).

Box 4
Clinical case, part 4

Noah's initial laboratory tests were all within normal range, and he was negative for HIV and other STIs. He reported 90% adherence at the first visit, approximately 6 weeks after initiating PrEP, and had no new partners at that time. He then missed his 3-month appointment but communicated through the portal to explain that he was busy at work and had not missed any doses. He was given a 1-month bridge prescription, and he made it to the laboratory the next week. He remained HIV negative for the following year, with normal renal function. He then missed an appointment but left a message to say he decided to stop PrEP. He did not like taking a pill every day and he was no longer in a relationship. He and Meredith broke up, and he was not having sex with anyone. He thought he was low risk, and it was too inconvenient to get to the clinic.

Clinical reasons to discontinue PrEP include HIV infection or significant renal impairment (CrCl<60 mL/min for TDF/FTC and glomerular filtration rate <15 mL/min for TAF/FTC). These individuals should be evaluated for other possible causes of renal impairment and monitored. A positive HIV test for anyone receiving PrEP should prompt immediate supplemental diagnostic testing, HIV genotype testing, intensification of the antiretroviral regimen, and referral to an experienced HIV provider. Intensification can quickly be accomplished via the addition of a third antiretroviral drug to TDF/FTC or TAF/FTC chosen in consultation with an HIV specialist, even if the individual will be transitioning to another practitioner. This approach facilitates rapid viral suppression, possibly reducing the risk of further transmission, formation of viral reservoirs, and immune system damage.[55–57] Patients with confirmed or suspected HIV should be counseled that acute infection increases the risk of transmission.

Follow-up remains important for patients who choose to discontinue PrEP for nonclinical reasons. HIV protection wanes over 7 to 10 days. Practitioners should document the most recent HIV status and reported adherence, the reason for stopping, and known risks at the time of discontinuation. If an individual has been off PrEP for more than 1 week and then wishes to resume, initial assessments should be repeated (see **Table 1**).

Nonoccupational Postexposure Prophylaxis

As with PrEP, nurses of all levels can participate in making needed medications available. Because nPEP regimens are dictated by clinical practice guidelines, standing order sets can be used for RN-led nPEP care. O'Byrne and colleagues[58] report on the successful implementation of an RN-led nPEP program in Canada. In the case of Noah (**Box 5**), he needs to be on nPEP, because PrEP does not offer protection once an exposure has occurred.

> **Box 5**
> **Clinical case, part 5**
>
> Five months later, Noah calls asking for a same-day appointment. Two nights ago, he cohosted a party, drank too much, and had receptive, condomless anal intercourse with a man he met that night. The following day a mutual friend texted Noah and asked if his "hookup" had revealed that he is HIV positive. Noah has a few of his PrEP pills left and asks if he should start them.

It is essential to build functional systems for patients to access nPEP. Yankellow and Yingling[59] describe the numerous systemic issues that need to be addressed for effective provision of nPEP. When needed, nPEP should be started as soon as possible and within 72 hours of sexual or injection exposure. Therefore, the nurse should ensure that all clinical staff are aware the service is available, payment assistance programs are in place in case they are needed, and local pharmacies stock the medication 7 d/wk.

Current approved agents and regimens

The WHO (2016), CDC (2016), and the Canadian Institutes of Health Research HIV Trials Network[60] all offer clinical practice guidelines for nPEP (**Table 2**). All regimens are based on 3-drug combination therapy, using 2 nucleoside reverse transcriptase inhibitors (typically TDF/FTC) and an additional antiretroviral (typically an integrase inhibitor or protease inhibitor). All the guidelines recommend a 28-day course of treatment. Because the 3 clinical practice guidelines vary considerably in selection of antiretroviral agents, this article does not provide explicit prescribing guidance. Instead, the authors recommend that nurses consult source guidelines within their jurisdictions. In addition, nurses in the United States should be aware that the CDC operates a PEP hotline for no-cost clinician consultations (1-888-448-4911).

Table 2
Nonoccupational postexposure prophylaxis regimens for adults and adolescents with normal renal function

	WHO[61]	CDC[62]	Canadian[60,63]
Preferred	TDF/lamivudine or TDF/FTC and lopinavir/ritonavir or atazanavir/ritonavir	TDF/FTC and raltegravir or dolutegravir	TDF/FTC and darunavir/ritonavir or dolutegravir or raltegravir
Alternative	TDF/lamivudine or TDF/FTC and raltegravir or darunavir/ritonavir or efavirenz	TDF/FTC and darunavir/ritonavir	zidovudine/lamivudine or TDF/lamivudine and atazanavir/ritonavir or darunavir/cobicistat or elvitegravir/cobicistat or lopinavir/ritonavir

Data from Refs.[60–62]

Patient identification

nPEP is indicated for the urgent prevention of HIV, and identification of candidate patients is an essential component of an nPEP program. Determining whether a patient is a candidate for nPEP requires knowledge of the type of exposure and information about the source patient's HIV status. Absent the ability to confirm that the source patient does not have HIV, an individual who had a possible HIV exposure during higher-risk activities (**Table 3**) should be offered nPEP. In a situation in which a source is known to have HIV with persistently undetectable viral load, nPEP is not indicated (U = U). However, confirmation of another person's persistently undetectable viral load is often difficult, and it is ultimately the patient's choice whether to take nPEP.

Table 3 Determining whether nonoccupational postexposure prophylaxis is indicated	
	Is nPEP Indicated?
Lower-risk Exposure	
• Oral-vaginal contact • Oral-anal contact • Oral-penile contact	nPEP not indicated unless: • Open sores in mouth or vagina, anus, or penis • Gum disease with oral exposure • Source is HIV+ with high viral load • Blood exposure
Higher-risk Exposure	
• Receptive or insertive vaginal or anal intercourse • Needle sharing • Injuries with exposure to blood or other bodily fluid	nPEP indicated if HIV+ partner without persistently undetectable viral load or HIV status unknown
Consult nPEP Guideline or call CDC PEP hotline: 1-888-448-4911	

Data from NYSDOH AIDS Institute. PEP for Non-Occupational Exposure to HIV (NPEP). New York City; 2018.

Access and follow-up

To reduce the risk of HIV infection, nPEP should be started as soon as possible after a higher-risk exposure, and generally no later than 72 hours after the exposure. Before initiating nPEP, baseline laboratory tests are needed (see **Table 1**). Treatment should not be delayed while awaiting these laboratory results. Although many pharmacies routinely stock the antiretrovirals that are part of the nPEP regimens, the nurse or clinic staff should phone ahead to ensure that the medications are on hand. If the pharmacy is unable to dispense a full 28-day supply of each medication, a 2-day to 3-day supply should be dispensed to allow time to procure the remaining doses.

Follow-up during and after nPEP treatment is essential to promote adherence, monitor treatment, screen for infections, and rule out HIV seroconversion. Initial follow-up for adherence can be via phone or telehealth strategies. These initial follow-up interactions should focus on confirming the patient has started the regimen and is tolerating it. Treatment monitoring with additional laboratory testing (ie, renal and hepatic function testing) is only indicated in patients whose underlying health warrants such monitoring. Screening for HIV and other infections should be done at baseline and as needed thereafter, with a confirmatory HIV test performed 1 month and 3 months after the exposure. After completing a month of nPEP, patients who continue to be at risk for HIV infection should be transitioned to PrEP (**Box 6**).

> **Box 6**
> **Clinical case, part 6**
>
> When contacted, Noah's recent sex partner was transparent in explaining that he has been positive for 15 years, is adherent with his antiretroviral therapy, and his viral load has been undetectable for years. The new partner acknowledged that he probably should have revealed his status, and they should have used a condom, but that everything he has read indicates that his risk of transmitting HIV to a partner is low, if not nonexistent. Using a patient portal on his phone, the + partner even shared month-old laboratory results to Noah. Although Noah understands that he is at low risk of contracting HIV, he is concerned that the partner's viral load could have increased if he had stopped his medication since these last laboratory tests. Noah decides to take nPEP for a month and then transition back to PrEP.

The nurse should draw the laboratory tests indicated for PrEP (which include tests for nPEP) and start Noah on nPEP for the prevention of HIV. After a month, if Noah is HIV negative, his drug regimen can be deintensified and he can continue on PrEP. Alternatively, Noah could use event-driven PrEP if he has infrequent exposures that he is able to plan at least 2 hours in advance. Although there is good evidence that it is effective,[36] as mentioned previously, event-driven PrEP is off label in the United States and Canada and has only been studied in MSM.

SUMMARY

With a global presence throughout all elements of the health care system, nurses are uniquely positioned to prevent new HIV infections. Across all settings of care, nurses can educate clients about strategies to prevent HIV infection, including pharmacoprevention. For people with risk for HIV, nurses can prescribe or furnish PrEP. For people with a possible HIV exposure, nurses can facilitate access to nPEP. These 2 strategies, along with TasP, can effectively eliminate new HIV infections in this generation.

DISCLOSURE

The authors have nothing to disclose.

REFERENCES

1. Achan J, Talisuna AO, Erhart A, et al. Quinine, an old anti-malarial drug in a modern world: Role in the treatment of malaria. Malar J 2011;10:1–12.
2. Connor EM, Sperling RS, Gelber R, et al. Reduction of Maternal-Infant Transmission of Human Immunodeficiency Virus Type 1 with Zidovudine Treatment. N Engl J Med 1994;331(18):1173–80.
3. Cardo DM, Culver DH, Ciesielski CA, et al. A Case-Control Study of HIV Seroconversion in Health Care Workers After Percutaneous Exposure. N Engl J Med 1997; 337(21):1485–90.
4. United States Public Health Service. Public Health Service guidelines for the management of health-care worker exposures to HIV and recommendations for postexposure prophylaxis. Centers for Disease Control and Prevention. MMWR Recomm Rep 1998;47(RR-7):1–33.
5. World Health Organization. Antiretroviral drugs for treating pregnant women and preventing HIV infections in infants: towards universal access (2006 version). Geneva (Switzerland): WHO Press; 2006. p. 1–92.

6. Rowland C. An HIV treatment cost taxpayers millions. The government patented it. But a pharma giant is making billions. The Washington Post 2019.

7. Cohen MS, Chen YQ, McCauley M, et al. Antiretroviral therapy for the prevention of HIV-1 transmission. N Engl J Med 2016;375(9):830–9.

8. Bavinton BR, Pinto AN, Phanuphak N, et al. Viral suppression and HIV transmission in serodiscordant male couples: An international, prospective, observational, cohort study. Lancet 2019;5(1):e348–447.

9. Rodger AJ, Cambiano V, Phillips AN, et al. Risk of HIV transmission through condomless sex in serodifferent gay couples with the HIV-positive partner taking suppressive antiretroviral therapy (PARTNER): final results of a multicentre, prospective, observational study. Lancet 2019;393(10189):2428–38.

10. Rodger AJ, Cambiano V, Bruun T, et al. Sexual activity without condoms and risk of HIV transmission in serodifferent couples when the HIV-positive partner is using suppressive antiretroviral therapy. JAMA 2016;316(2):171–81.

11. Centers for Disease Control and Prevention. HIV Among Hispanics/Latinos in the United States and Dependent Areas. HIV/Statistics. 2015;17(November): Available at: http://www.cdc.gov/hiv/group/racialethnic/hispanic. Accessed December 23, 2019.

12. Goldstein RH, Streed CG, Cahill S. Being PrEPared-Preexposure Prophylaxis and HIV Disparities. N Engl J Med 2018;379(14):1293–5.

13. Centers for Disease Control and Prevention. HIV Risk and Prevention. HIV/AIDS. 2016. Available at: https://www.cdc.gov/hiv/risk/.

14. Centers for Disease Control and Prevention. Preexposure prophylaxis for the prevention of HIV infection in the United States - 2017 update: a clinical practice guideline. Atlanta (GA): Centers for Disease Control and Prevention; 2017. https://doi.org/10.1016/S0040-4039(01)91800-3.

15. Centers for Disease Control and Prevention. Updated guidelines for postexposure prophylaxis After sexual, injection drug, or other nonoccupational exposures to HIV-United States, 2016. Washington, DC: Centers for Disease Control and Prevention; 2016.

16. Roland ME, Neilands TB, Krone MR, et al. Seroconversion Following Nonoccupational Postexposure Prophylaxis against HIV. Clin Infect Dis 2005;41(10):1507–13.

17. World Health Organization. Guidelines on post-exposure prophylaxis for HIV and the use of Co-trimoxazole prophylaxis for HIV-related infections among adults, adolescents and children: recommendations for a public health approach. Geneva (Switzerland): Gene; 2014.

18. World Health Organization. Guidance on pre-exposure oral prophylaxis (PrEP) for serodiscordant couples, men and transgender women who have sex with men at high risk of HIV: recommendations for use in the context of demonstration projects. Geneva (Switzerland): WHO Press; 2012. https://doi.org/10.1162/leon_r_00510.

19. Owens DK, Davidson KW, Krist AH, et al. Preexposure prophylaxis for the prevention of HIV infection: US preventive services task force recommendation statement. JAMA 2019;321(22):2203–13.

20. United States Food and Drug Administration. Tenofovir alafenamide/emtricitabine prescribing information. 2019. Available at: https://www.accessdata.fda.gov/drugsatfda_docs/label/2016/208215s000lbl.pdf. Accessed December 23, 2019.

21. Centers for Disease Control and Prevention. Estimated HIV incidence and prevalence in the United States, 2010–2016. vol. 24. Atlanta (GA): Centers for Disease Control and Prevention; 2019.

22. Centers for Disease Control and Prevention. HIV prevention pill not reaching most Americans who could benefit-especially people of color. National Center for HIV/AIDS, Viral Hepatitis, STD, and TB Prevention. Atlanta (GA): Centers for Disease Control and Prevention; 2018. Available at: https://www.cdc.gov/nchhstp/newsroom/2018/croi-2018-PrEP-press-release.html.

23. Golub SA. NYSDOH AI GOALS framework for sexual history taking in primary care. New York: New York State Department of Health; 2019.

24. Centers for Disease Control and Prevention. Taking a sexual history. Atlanta (GA): Centers for Disease Control and Prevention; 2011.

25. Smith D, Yi Pan C, Pals S, et al. A brief screening tool to assess the risk of contracting HIV infection among active injection drug users. J Addict Med 2015;9(3):226-32.

26. NYSDOH AIDS Institute. PrEP to prevent HIV and promote sexual health. New York: New York State Department of Health; 2019. Available at: https://cdn.hivguidelines.org/wp-content/uploads/20191023094009/NYSDOH-AI-PrEP-to-Prevent-HIV-and-Promote-Sexual-Health_10-23-2019_HG.pdf.

27. O'Byrne P. Human Immunodeficiency Virus Preexposure Prophylaxis: A Quick Guide for Primary Care Practice. J Nurse Pract 2019;15(8):564–7.

28. Haider A, Adler RR, Schneider E, et al. Assessment of Patient-Centered Approaches to Collect Sexual Orientation and Gender Identity Information in the Emergency Department. JAMA Netw Open 2018;1(8):e186506.

29. GLMA. Guidelines for the care of lesbian, gay, bisexual, and transgender patients. Washington, DC: Gay and Lesbian Medical Association; 2006. Available at: http://glma.org/_data/n_0001/resources/live/GLMA guidelines 2006 FINAL.pdf.

30. Cotler K, Yingling C, Broholm C. Preventing New Human Immunodeficiency Virus Infections With Pre-exposure Prophylaxis. J Nurse Pract 2018;14(5):376–82.

31. Traeger MW, Schroeder SE, Wright EJ, et al. Effects of Pre-exposure Prophylaxis for the Prevention of Human Immunodeficiency Virus Infection on Sexual Risk Behavior in Men Who Have Sex with Men: A Systematic Review and Meta-analysis. Clin Infect Dis 2018;67(5):676–86.

32. Jenness SM, Weiss KM, Goodreau SM, et al. Incidence of gonorrhea and chlamydia following human immunodeficiency virus preexposure prophylaxis among men who have sex with men: A modeling study. Clin Infect Dis 2017;65(5):712–8.

33. United States Food and Drug Administration. FDA approves second drug to prevent HIV infection as part of ongoing efforts to end the HIV epidemic | FDA. FDA News Release 2019. Available at: https://www.fda.gov/news-events/press-announcements/fda-approves-second-drug-prevent-hiv-infection-part-ongoing-efforts-end-hiv-epidemic. Accessed October 6, 2019.

34. WHO. What'S the 2+1+1? Event-driven oral pre-exposure prophylaxis to prevent HIV for men who have sex with men: update to WHO'S recommendation on oral prep. Geneva (Switzerland): WHO Press; 2019.

35. Saag MS, Benson CA, Gandhi RT, et al. Antiretroviral drugs for treatment and prevention of HIV infection in adults: 2018 recommendations of the international antiviral society-USA panel. JAMA 2018;320(4):379–96.

36. Molina J-M, Capitant C, Spire B, et al. On-Demand Preexposure Prophylaxis in Men at High Risk for HIV-1 Infection. N Engl J Med 2015;373(23):2237–46.

37. Johnson J. The HIV PrEP and microbicides pipeline. New York: Treatment Action Group; 2018.

38. BHIVA/BASHH. Guidelines on the use of HIV pre-exposure prophylaxis (PrEP). Hertfordshire (UK): British HIV Association; 2018.

39. O'Byrne P, MacPherson P, Orser L, et al. Clinical Considerations and Protocols for Nurse-Led PrEP. J Assoc Nurses AIDS Care 2019;30(3):301–11.
40. NYSDOH AIDS Institute. PrEP to prevent HIV and promote sexual health. New York: New York State Department of Health; 2019.
41. World Health Organization. WHO implementation tool for pre-exposure prophylaxis (PrEP) of HIV infection. Geneva (Switzerland): WHO Press; 2017.
42. Gupta SK, Post FA, Arribas JR, et al. Renal safety of tenofovir alafenamide vs. tenofovir disoproxil fumarate: A pooled analysis of 26 clinical trials. AIDS 2019; 33(9):1455–65.
43. NIH. Antiretroviral Drug Use in Pregnant Women with HIV: Pharmacokinetic and Toxicity Data in Human Pregnancy and Recommendations for Use in Pregnancy. 2019. Available at: https://aidsinfo.nih.gov/guidelines/htmltables/3/7509. Accessed December 23, 2019.
44. WHO. WHO technical brief: preventing HIV during pregnancy and breastfeeding in the context of PrEP. WHO/HIV/2017.09. Geneva (Switzerland): WHO Tech Br; 2017.
45. Mikati T, Jamison K, Daskalakis DC. Immediate PrEP Initiation at New York City Sexual Health Clinics. In: Conference on Retroviruses and Opportunistic Infections. Seattle, WA, March 4, 2019.
46. Kamis KF, Marx GE, Scott KA, et al. Same-Day HIV Pre-Exposure Prophylaxis (PrEP) Initiation During Drop-in Sexually Transmitted Diseases Clinic Appointments Is a Highly Acceptable, Feasible, and Safe Model that Engages Individuals at Risk for HIV into PrEP Care. Open Forum Infect Dis 2019;6(7):1–7.
47. Glidden DV, Amico KR, Liu AY, et al. Symptoms, Side Effects and Adherence in the iPrEx Open-Label Extension. Clin Infect Dis 2016;62(9):1172–7.
48. Hiransuthikul A, Janamnuaysook R, Himmad K, et al. Drug-drug interactions between feminizing hormone therapy and pre-exposure prophylaxis among transgender women: the iFACT study. J Int AIDS Soc 2019;22(7):e25338.
49. Sidebottom D, Ekström AM, Strömdahl S. A systematic review of adherence to oral pre-exposure prophylaxis for HIV - How can we improve uptake and adherence? BMC Infect Dis 2018;18(1):1–14.
50. Chu M, Cotler K, Yingling C. Understanding patient motivations for HIV pre-exposure prophylaxis initiation and adherence. J Am Assoc Nurse Pract 2019. https://doi.org/10.1097/jxx.0000000000000282.
51. Centers for Disease Control and Prevention. HIV/AIDS: HIV Cost effectiveness. 2014. Available at: http://www.cdc.gov/hiv/prevention/ongoing/costeffectiveness/. Accessed December 23, 2019.
52. Van Der Helm JJ, Hoebe CJPA, Van Rooijen MS, et al. High performance and acceptability of self-collected rectal swabs for diagnosis of Chlamydia trachomatis and Neisseria gonorrhoeae in men who have sex with men and women. Sex Transm Dis 2009;36(8):493–7.
53. Schoeman SA, Stewart CMW, Booth RA, et al. Assessment of best single sample for finding chlamydia in women with and without symptoms: A diagnostic test study. BMJ 2012;345(7887):1–17.
54. Seidmana D, Webera S, CarlsonKimberly Witt J. Family planning providers' role in offering PrEP to women. Contraception 2018;97(6):467–70.
55. AIDSinfo. Panel on Antiretroviral Guidelines for Adults and Adolescents. Guidelines for the Use of Antiretroviral Agents in Adults and Adolescents with HIV. Dep Heal Hum Serv. 298. 2018. Available at: https://aidsinfo.nih.gov/contentfiles/lvguidelines/adultandadolescentgl.pdf. Accessed December 23, 2019.

56. Coffey S, Bacchetti P, Sachdev D, et al. RAPID antiretroviral therapy: high virologic suppression rates with immediate antiretroviral therapy initiation in a vulnerable urban clinic population. AIDS 2019;33(5):825–32.

57. Smith DK, Switzer WM, Peters P, et al. A strategy for PrEP clinicians to manage ambiguous HIV test results during follow-up visits. Open Forum Infect Dis 2018;5(8):1–6.

58. O'Byrne P, Macpherson P, Roy M, et al. Overviewing a nurse-led, community-based HIV PEP program: Applying the extant literature in frontline practice. Public Health Nurs 2014;32(3):256–65.

59. Yankellow I, Yingling CT. Nonoccupational Postexposure Prophylaxis: An Essential Tool for HIV Prevention. J Nurse Pract 2019;15(10):764–71.

60. Tan D, Hull M, Yoong D, et al. Canadian guideline on HIV pre-exposure prophylaxis and nonoccupational postexposure prophylaxis. Can Med Assoc J 2017;189(47):E1448-58.

61. WHO. Consolidated Guidelines on the Use of Antiretroviral Drugs for Treating and Preventing HIV Infection. 2016. http://apps.who.int/iris/bitstream/10665/85322/1/WHO_HIV_2013.7_eng.pdf. Accessed January 2, 2020.

62. Centers for Disease Control and Prevention. Updated guidelines for postexposure prophylaxis after sexual, injection drug, or other nonoccupational exposures to HIV-United States, Centers for Disease Control and Prevention; 2016. Washington, DC: 2016. Available at: https://www.cdc.gov/hiv/pdf/programresources/cdc-hiv-npep-guidelines.pdf.

63. NYSDOH AIDS Institute. PEP for non-occupational exposure to HIV (NPEP). New York: New York State Department of Health; 2018.

Sexually Transmitted Infections and Human Immunodeficiency Virus

Robin M. Lawson, DNP, CRNP, ACNP-BC, NP-C

KEYWORDS

- Human immunodeficiency virus • Sexually transmitted infections • Transmission
- Acquisition • Infectiousness • Susceptibility

KEY POINTS

- The human immunodeficiency virus (HIV) and sexually transmitted infections (STIs) are considered epidemics in the United States.
- Research on the association between STIs and HIV infectiousness and susceptibility has shown that STIs promote HIV acquisition and transmission.
- Early diagnosis and treatment of both HIV and STIs is essential to ending these associated epidemics.

INTRODUCTION

The human immunodeficiency virus (HIV) and sexually transmitted infections (STIs) are considered epidemics in the United States. More than a million individuals were living with HIV in the United States at the end of 2017,[1] and 37,832 individuals were newly diagnosed in 2018.[2] The prevalence of HIV diagnosis in the United States in 2018 by sex and transmission category is shown in **Fig. 1** (men) and **Fig. 2** (women). Most newly diagnosed cases occur in men who have sex with men (MSM).[2] About 80% of new HIV transmissions result from individuals who do not know they are infected or are not receiving consistent care.[3] Delayed HIV diagnoses in at-risk populations remain substantial and hinder entry to early care to decrease adverse health outcomes and reduce the risk of HIV transmission.[4]

Almost 20 million new STIs are diagnosed annually in the United States, with about half occurring in young women and men who are 15 to 24 years of age.[5] Because some STIs are frequently asymptomatic and not diagnosed, STI prevalence is underestimated.[6] MSM are highly susceptible to STIs,[2,7] particularly if they do not use condoms during casual anal intercourse.[8,9] This article focuses on common STIs that are

Capstone College of Nursing, The University of Alabama, 650 University Boulevard, East, Tuscaloosa, AL 35401, USA
E-mail address: rmlawson@ua.edu

Nurs Clin N Am 55 (2020) 445–456
https://doi.org/10.1016/j.cnur.2020.06.007
0029-6465/20/© 2020 Elsevier Inc. All rights reserved.

nursing.theclinics.com

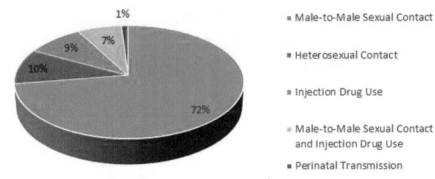

Fig. 1. Prevalence of HIV infection in the United States by transmission category for men and boys aged 13 years and older. (*Data from* Centers for Disease Control and Prevention. HIV surveillance report, 2018 [Preliminary]; vol. 30. Available at: http://www.cdc.gov/hiv/library/reports/hiv-surveillance.html. Published November, 2019. Accessed January 18, 2020.)

more frequently associated with HIV infection, such as chlamydia, gonorrhea, syphilis, and herpes simplex virus (HSV).

RELATIONSHIP BETWEEN SEXUALLY TRANSMITTED INFECTIONS AND HUMAN IMMUNODEFICIENCY VIRUS TRANSMISSION

Research has shown that individuals who have STIs are more prone to HIV acquisition.[10–13] HIV is particularly affected by accompanying common viral or bacterial STIs associated with mucosal inflammation and genital ulcers.[14] With inflammation or skin integrity disruption, HIV transmission can occur more easily by increasing the infectiousness of the individual infected, the susceptibility of the partner, or both.[12] Behaviors that increase the risk of acquiring one infection frequently increase the risk of acquiring other infections.[10] Whether engaging in oral, anal, or vaginal intercourse, behaviors that increase the risk of acquiring HIV and STIs include having multiple partners, having anonymous partners, using alcohol or drugs, and not wearing condoms.[10] This article highlights the role genital tract inflammation plays in the relationship between STIs and HIV transmission.

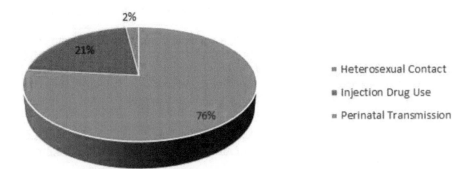

Fig. 2. Prevalence of HIV infection in the United States by transmission category for women and girls aged 13 years and older. (*Data from* Centers for Disease Control and Prevention. HIV surveillance report, 2018 [Preliminary]; vol. 30. Available at: http://www.cdc.gov/hiv/library/reports/hiv-surveillance.html. Published November, 2019. Accessed January 18, 2020.)

- Research on the association between STIs and HIV infectiousness and susceptibility has shown that STIs promote HIV acquisition and transmission via inflammation and ulceration.[13] STIs that cause ulcerations, such as syphilis and HSV-2, break down the mucosal integrity and recruit activated target cells that contain an enriched group of cells that carry cluster of differentiation 4 (CD4) cell receptors. The lesions develop proinflammatory cytokines that then cause an increased number of inflammatory cells in the genital tract environment that augment HIV in vivo replication.[13] STIs may also increase the expression of HIV-binding ligands that promote HIV acquisition and transmission.[13] Further, although STIs that cause ulcers are linked to the highest rates of HIV susceptibility, STIs that cause inflammation (chlamydia and gonorrhea) also facilitate inflammatory cell recruitment and increase the likelihood of acquiring and transmitting HIV.[13]
- The female genital mucosa is an essential physical and biological barrier that serves as the first line of defense against HIV and other invading microorganisms.[15] STI pathogen pattern recognition, by receptors expressed on either the inside or surface of the cell, causes the mucosal barrier to become inflamed.[15] Depending on the STI, a variety of mucosal responses, such as ulcers and discharge, can occur in an effort to get rid of the invading microorganism. These responses pathologically disrupt the barrier and intensify the ability for HIV to gain access to submucosal target cells.[15] In addition, instinctive responses to STIs can cause an increase in the number of immune cells, including those that are main targets of HIV, and may play a significant role in the connection between STIs and a heightened susceptibility to HIV acquisition.[15]
- Bamniya and colleagues[16] conducted a cross-sectional study on the prevalence of lower genital tract infections in women who were HIV positive. Results revealed that lower genital tract infections were more prevalent in HIV-positive women (36%) compared with HIV-negative women (24%). A significantly higher number of genital tract infections was found in HIV-positive patients with CD4 cell counts less than 200/mm^3. These researchers concluded that the vaginal ecosystem is altered in the presence of lower genital tract infections and thereby increases the risk of acquiring opportunistic pathogens.[16]

Gonorrhea, Chlamydia, and Human Immunodeficiency Virus

Chlamydia (*Chlamydia trachomatis*) is the most common notifiable STI in the United States and occurs twice as often in women than in men.[6] More than 1.7 million chlamydia cases were reported in 2017.[6] **Fig. 3** shows the reported chlamydia cases by sex and age groups for individuals aged 15 to 64 years. Chlamydia may be asymptomatic, but it is an inflammatory infection that has been shown to be linked to a higher risk for acquiring HIV.[17–19]

The second most common notifiable STI in the United States is gonorrhea (*Neisseria gonorrhoeae)*. More than half a million gonorrhea cases were reported in 2017.[6] **Fig. 4** shows the reported gonorrhea cases by sex and age groups for individuals aged 15 to 64 years. Gonorrhea rates have been increasing in recent years,[5] and have increased most dramatically among MSM.[6] Gonorrhea is also an inflammatory infection that has been linked to a higher risk of acquiring HIV.[18–20] The studies discussed here highlight recent findings related to gonorrhea, chlamydia, and HIV infection.

- Buckner and colleagues[17] developed one of the first endocervical models for in vitro study of the interactions between chlamydia and HIV. Results of the study suggest that chlamydia-infected endocervical epithelial cells could promote not

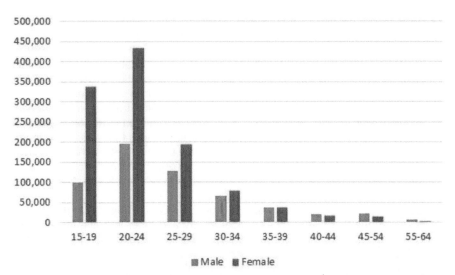

Fig. 3. Reported chlamydia cases by sex and age groups in the United States in 2017 for individuals aged 15 to 64 years. (*Data from* Centers for Disease Control and Prevention. Sexually transmitted disease surveillance 2017. Atlanta: U.S. Department of Health and Human Services; 2018. Available at: https://www.cdc.gov/std/stats17/2017-STD-Surveillance-Report_CDC-clearance-9.10.18.pdf.)

only HIV migration across the mucosal barrier but also subsequent replication or infection in underlying target cells.[17]

• Adachi and colleagues[18] investigated gonorrhea and chlamydia prevalence and the connection between HIV mother-to-child transmission (MTCT). A total of 249

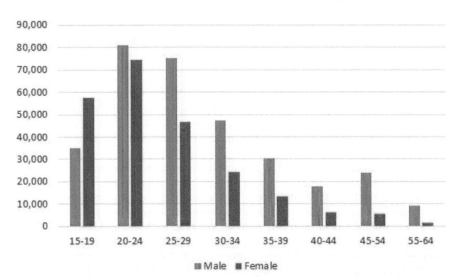

Fig. 4. Reported gonorrhea cases by sex and age groups in the United States in 2017 for individuals aged 15 to 64 years. (*Data from* Centers for Disease Control and Prevention. Sexually transmitted disease surveillance 2017. Atlanta: U.S. Department of Health and Human Services; 2018. Available at: https://www.cdc.gov/std/stats17/2017-STD-Surveillance-Report_CDC-clearance-9.10.18.pdf.)

(18.1%) women tested positive for chlamydia, 63 (4.6%) tested positive for gonorrhea, and 35 (2.5%) tested positive for both chlamydia and gonorrhea. Of the 117 (8.5%) cases of HIV MTCT, the lowest rate of transmission was shown to be among the infants born to mothers not infected with gonorrhea and chlamydia (8.1%) compared with those who were positive for only chlamydia (10.7%) and both gonorrhea and chlamydia (14.3%). Infants born to mothers who were infected with chlamydia had nearly a 1.5-fold greater risk for acquiring HIV. Adachi and colleagues[18] concluded that the pregnant women who were HIV positive were at high risk for being gonorrhea and chlamydia positive. In addition, a higher risk of HIV MTCT is possible in HIV-infected pregnant women who are also infected with gonorrhea and chlamydia.[18]

- Taylor and colleagues[19] reviewed the HIV-positive status and HIV viral loads (VLs) in men who were diagnosed with rectal chlamydia and gonorrhea to assess the potential risk of HIV transmission and acquisition. Of the 1591 men who were tested during the 2-year study period, 506 (31.8%) tested positive for rectal gonorrhea, chlamydia, or both, and 119 (23.5%) were also infected with HIV.[19] The mean VL was greater in men coinfected with HIV and rectal gonorrhea/chlamydia compared with men diagnosed only with HIV.[19] More than 50% of the HIV-infected men who were positive for gonorrhea or chlamydia were found to have detectable VL collected within 1 year of the rectal testing time, showing the HIV transmission risk.[19]

Syphilis and Human Immunodeficiency Virus

Syphilis is caused by *Treponema pallidum*, a bacterium that creates genital ulcers.[6] Almost 31,000 primary or secondary syphilis cases were reported in the United States in 2017.[6] **Fig. 5** shows the reported primary or secondary syphilis cases by sex and age groups for individuals aged 15 to 64 years. Syphilis rates have increased in recent years,[5] and have increased most dramatically among MSM.[6] Coinfection of HIV and syphilis has been found to exist frequently in MSM,[6,9,10] and is associated with an increased risk of HIV transmission.[9] A recent increase in congenital syphilis has also been reported,[6,21] which has been attributed to an increase in syphilis among reproductive-age women.[6] The 2 studies discussed here highlight recent findings related to the association between syphilis and HIV.

- Taylor and colleagues[22] examined VLs among HIV-infected individuals diagnosed with primary and secondary syphilis. More than 50% of the HIV-infected individuals who were subsequently diagnosed with syphilis had VLs detected within 6 months of being diagnosed with syphilis. This finding supports virologic and behavioral risk for transmitting HIV to others.[22]
- Marcus and colleagues[9] conducted a study on risk factors for HIV and STI diagnosis among MSM. Most men were reportedly being tested (61%) because of unprotected anal intercourse (UAI). Results revealed that there was a strong association between UAI and a diagnosis of HIV. In addition, a syphilis diagnosis was strongly associated with a diagnosis of HIV.[9]

Herpes Simplex Virus Type 2 and Human Immunodeficiency Virus

Although HSV is not a nationally notifiable STI in the United States,[6] it is one of the most prevalent.[5] HSV-2 is a lifelong infection [23] that may present as painful ulcers in the genital area and is associated with high morbidity and mortality of infected neonates.[24] HSV-2 is often associated with HIV.[10,12,23,25–27] The studies discussed here highlight recent findings related to HSV-2 and HIV infection.

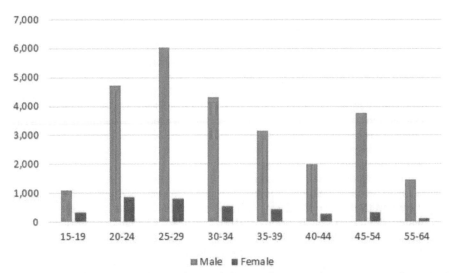

Fig. 5. Reported primary and secondary syphilis cases by sex and age groups in the United States in 2017 for individuals aged 15 to 64 years. (*Data from* Centers for Disease Control and Prevention. Sexually transmitted disease surveillance 2017. Atlanta: U.S. Department of Health and Human Services; 2018. Available at: https://www.cdc.gov/std/stats17/2017-STD-Surveillance-Report_CDC-clearance-9.10.18.pdf.)

- Keller and colleagues[25] tested the hypothesis that HIV and HSV-2 dual infection is associated with vaginal dysbiosis and/or cervicovaginal inflammation. Results of the 12-week study revealed an increase in diverse anaerobes and a decrease in *Lactobacillus crispatus* when comparing HIV-1$^+$/HSV-2$^+$ with HIV-1$^-$/HSV-2$^-$ women. Genital HSV outbreaks were found to be more numerous for HIV$^+$ versus HIV$^-$ women. Keller and colleagues[25] concluded that increased cervicovaginal inflammation and microbial variability in HSV-2 and HIV dually infected women may detrimentally affect the health of the genital tract and, without antiretroviral therapy, promote HIV shedding.
- Looker and colleagues[23] conducted a systematic review and meta-analysis on the effect of HSV-2 infection on HIV acquisition. HIV acquisition was about tripled in individuals who had established HSV-2 and was almost doubled in higher-risk populations. The highest risk of HIV acquisition was found to be in individuals who had recently acquired HSV-2. According to the findings, there is a strong indication for a biological effect of HSV-2 infection on HIV because the severity and frequency of ulceration in the genital area, shedding of the virus, and associated genital tract mucosal inflammation are highest in new HSV-2 infections and typically decrease over time. Such findings have major implications for the management of individuals with HSV-2 infection, particularly those who have been newly diagnosed.[23]
- Domercant and colleagues[26] examined the seroprevalence of HSV-2 among pregnant women. Results revealed the overall weighted prevalence to be 31.4% for HSV-2. In addition, the prevalence of HIV in women who were HSV-2 positive was 5 times higher than for those who were HSV-2 negative.[26]
- In the HIV Prevention Trials Network 071 (PopART) study, Bradley and colleagues[27] used HIV/HSV-2 serologic findings to examine the relationship between HIV and HSV-2. Almost 39,000 adults participated in the study. Results revealed a 6-fold higher odds of HIV infection among men and women infected with HSV-2.[27]

Sexually Transmitted Infections and Subsequent Human Immunodeficiency Virus Diagnosis

MSM are at high risk of HIV acquisition following the diagnosis of an STI.[28] The studies discussed here highlight additional findings regarding this risk.

- Katz and colleagues[28] evaluated HIV incidence among MSM after being diagnosed with a different STIs. The state incidence of HIV diagnosis among all MSM was estimated at 0.4 per 100 person-years. MSM were found to be at greatest risk of acquiring HIV following a diagnosis of rectal gonorrhea. Other preceding STI diagnoses, in order of prevalence, included early syphilis, urethral gonorrhea, rectal chlamydial infection, pharyngeal gonorrhea, late syphilis, and urethral chlamydia.[28]
- Kelley and colleagues[7] conducted a longitudinal study consisting of a cohort of white and black sexually active, HIV-negative MSM who participated in routine testing for HIV and STI and completed questionnaires regarding behaviors. Results revealed that the incidence rates for all STIs were high, particularly for black MSM. After controlling for behavioral risk, a significant link was shown between rectal STIs and subsequent HIV acquisition. MSM with a diagnosis of rectal STI on follow up were more than 2.5 times more likely to acquire HIV compared with MSM without a diagnosis of rectal STI.[7]

Additional Studies on Concomitant Sexually Transmitted Infections and Human Immunodeficiency Virus

Adachi and colleagues[20] conducted a retrospective, cross-sectional clinical trial substudy of 899 mother-infant pairs in which the mother was HIV positive. Results revealed the HIV-positive women to be at high risk for having at least 1 STI (chlamydia, gonorrhea, syphilis, or cytomegalovirus). Additional findings indicated that the risk of HIV MTCT is almost double in the presence of 1 or more STIs.[20]

Vasanthamoorthy and Balachandar[12] conducted a retrospective observational study on the prevalence and epidemiologic characteristics of STIs in HIV-positive individuals seeking outpatient treatment. Results revealed that STIs are highly prevalent among HIV-positive individuals. Most of the patients in the study presented with vaginal discharge or pelvic inflammatory disease (PID), and the most common ulcerative STI was herpes. The morphologic characteristics of the patients were similar to those of individuals who were not HIV positive. These results highlight the importance of early diagnosis and combined management strategies for STIs and HIV.[12]

Joseph Davey and colleagues[29] conducted a cross-sectional study of pregnant women presenting for their first prenatal visits to assess the prevalence and correlation of STIs. Of the 242 women included in the study, 44% were HIV positive. The percentage of cases representing any STI was higher for HIV-positive women (39%) compared with HIV-negative women (28%). More than 30% of those who tested positive were coinfected with more than 1 STI. The most common STIs were chlamydia, trichomonas, and gonorrhea, which signifies a high prevalence of STIs that are curable.[29]

SEXUALLY TRANSMITTED INFECTIONS, HUMAN IMMUNODEFICIENCY VIRUS, AND ANTIRETROVIRAL THERAPY

STIs potentiate the infectiousness of individuals who have HIV by means of increasing the concentration of the virus in the genital tract and by increasing the possibility for acquisition of HIV in individuals who are at risk for the infection.[14] Antiretroviral therapy

(ART) has been shown to significantly decrease HIV transmission.[14,30,31] The studies discussed here highlight recent findings related to STIs, HIV, and ART.

- Cohen and colleagues[14] recently conducted a review of studies on the relationship between HIV and STIs with particular attention to changes associated with the biological interactions since ART has become available. Results of the review revealed several important findings. First, ART decreases HIV infectiousness and eliminates HIV transmission despite the presence of concomitant STIs. Second, even though ART stops HIV transmission, it does not halt the recurrent shedding of HIV in genital secretions. Third, HIV shedding is increased in the presence of STIs, but the viral copies are most likely not able to replicate or infect. In addition, HIV acquisition is prevented with preexposure prophylaxis (PrEP) by using a highly active combination of tenofovir disoproxil fumarate and emtricitabine (TDF/FTC) despite concomitant STIs.[14]
- Werner and colleagues[8] conducted a meta-analysis using data from trials and observational studies pertaining to HIV PrEP. Studies of PrEP in MSM that reported incidence of STIs were identified, and 20 studies from 24 publications were included in the meta-analysis. During the study period, most of the studies reported that STI incidence and/or sexual behavior either decreased or remained stable. As reported by Werner and colleagues,[8] MSM need access to STI testing at close intervals. With STI monitoring and early treatment, PrEP may decrease HIV incidence and exert positive effects in reducing the burden of STIs.[8]
- Champredon and colleagues[30] conducted a systematic review and meta-analysis to examine the effect of STI coinfections on HIV VL among individuals on ART. Studies that reported differences in the rate of HIV transmission or in VLs between individuals receiving ART who either were or were not coinfected with a different STI were included in the study. The meta-analysis of HIV VLs among the individuals receiving treatment did not reveal a statistically significant effect of STI coinfection. On average, VLs were 0.11 log 10 higher among coinfected individuals versus those not coinfected. According to Champredon and colleagues,[30] it is, therefore, not likely that coinfection diminishes the efficacy of treatment as prevention. However, too few data exist to determine whether or not certain STIs present a greater risk.[30]
- de Melo and colleagues[31] conducted a study to evaluate the transmission risk of STIs and HIV. Study participants included 200 serodifferent couples who had been in a stable relationship for 3 months, with 1 being on ART. The individuals who were HIV positive (70% female; 30% male) had been followed at an HIV couple's clinic for a median time period of 4.5 years and receiving ART for 3 months preceding the study. Results revealed that 5 of the 200 study participants had seroconverted. Mean serum VLs were more increased in HIV transmitters compared with nontransmitters. STIs were significantly higher in couples where seroconversion occurred, with syphilis being the most prevalent. The existence of STIs and the length of time for undetectable HIV viremia were linked to HIV transmission. de Melo and colleagues[31] concluded that the main protective factor for not transmitting HIV was undetectable viremia.

IMPORTANCE OF SEXUALLY TRANSMITTED INFECTION TREATMENT TO REDUCE INFECTIOUSNESS AND SUSCEPTIBILITY

Not only are STIs prevalent, they are a major cause of morbidity and mortality.[12,32] Undiagnosed chlamydia infections among many young women pose a concern because of the associated risk of infertility.[5] In addition, STIs such as chlamydia and gonorrhea can result in detrimental outcomes such as PID, chronic pelvic pain, and ectopic pregnancy.[6] In addition, STI MTCT can cause serious harm to the neonate,[6,24] including prematurity, neonatal pneumonia, neonatal ophthalmia, developmental disabilities, and death.[6] The increased prevalence of STIs in HIV-positive individuals signifies the importance of susceptibility and infectivity cofactors in HIV acquisition and transmission and also emphasizes the importance of early diagnosis and treatment of STIs to control the acquisition and transmission of HIV.[12]

Because many STIs are asymptomatic, screening is essential in early detection and prevention.[33] Evidence shows that having symptoms that lead to an STI diagnosis occurs in only about a third of pregnant women.[29] Such findings indicate that a large percentage of these women are not diagnosed and treated for curable STIs.[29] Because HIV and STI acquisition are so closely linked, a need to improve the screening and identification processes for both exists in this population in order to reduce the potential risk of adverse health events for women and children.[29] In addition to identifying and screening, there is an increased need to treat curable STIs in pregnant women to reduce the risk of HIV MTCT.[18,20,29] Because MSM are highly susceptible to STIs[7] and also at high risk for HIV acquisition following the diagnosis of an STI,[28] strategies to reduce the risk is imperative in this population. Prompt evaluation of symptoms suggestive of STIs such as PID, vaginal discharge, urethritis, cervicitis, epididymitis, proctitis, genital ulcers, anogenital warts, and pharyngitis is warranted so that an accurate diagnosis can be made and empiric treatment can be provided in order to prevent complications and the potential for further transmission.[33]

Recommendations for reducing the risk of getting HIV and STIs include:

- Abstaining from oral, anal, and vaginal sex or having a mutually monogamous relationship with someone who is not infected
- Using a new condom throughout each sexual activity whether it is oral, anal, or vaginal[33]
- Engaging in sexual behaviors that are less risky
- Decreasing the number of sex partners
- Eliminating or limiting the use of alcohol and drugs before and during sex
- Having a discussion with a health care provider about being tested for HIV and STIs
- Asking a health care provider if preexposure or postexposure prophylaxis is recommended to prevent being infected with HIV[10]

MSM who ask to be tested for HIV should also be tested for bacterial STIs.[9] In addition, individuals who have been diagnosed with HIV and subsequently develop an STI should seek counseling about reducing their risk and reducing their sex partners' risk of acquiring the infections.[10]

SUMMARY

There is high prevalence of STIs in HIV-positive individuals. Susceptibility and infectivity cofactors are associated with increased HIV acquisition and transmission. Prompt diagnosis and treatment of STIs to control HIV acquisition and transmission is of utmost importance.[12] Behavior change to reduce risks is imperative to preventing adverse health outcomes.[10,33] These associated epidemics, with one stimulating the other, call attention to the compelling need to gain control of one so that the other can be controlled.

DISCLOSURE

The author has nothing to disclose.

REFERENCES

1. Centers for Disease Control and Prevention. HIV surveillance report, 2018 (preliminary) 2019. vol. 30. Available at: http://www.cdc.gov/hiv/library/reports/hiv-surveillance.html. Accessed January 18, 2020.
2. Centers for Disease Control and Prevention. HIV in the United States and dependent areas 2019. Available at: https://www.cdc.gov/hiv/pdf/statistics/overview/cdc-hiv-us-ataglance.pdf. Accessed January 17, 2019.
3. Zihao L, Purcell DW, Sansome SL, et al. Vital signs: HIV transmission along the continuum of care - United States, 2016. MMWR Morb Mortal Wkly Rep 2019; 68(11):267–72.
4. Dailey AF, Hoots BE, Hall HI, et al. Vital signs: human immunodeficiency virus testing and diagnosis delays - United States. MMWR Morb Mortal Wkly Rep 2017;66(47):1300–6.
5. Satterwhite CL, Torrone E, Meites E, et al. Sexually transmitted infections among US women and men: prevalence and incidence estimates, 2008. Sex Transm Dis 2013;40(3):187–93.
6. Centers for Disease Control and Prevention. Sexually transmitted disease surveillance 2017. Atlanta (GA): U.S. Department of Health and Human Services; 2018. Available at: https://stacks.cdc.gov/view/cdc/59237. Accessed January 18, 2020.
7. Kelley CF, Vaughan AS, Luisi N, et al. The effect of high rates of bacterial sexually transmitted infections on HIV incidence in a cohort of black and white men who have sex with men in Atlanta, Georgia. AIDS Res Hum Retroviruses 2015;31(6): 587–92.
8. Werner RN, Gaskins M, Nast A, et al. Incidence of sexually transmitted infections in men who have sex with men and who are at substantial risk of HIV infection - A meta-analysis of data from trials and observational studies of HIV pre-exposure prophylaxis. PLoS One 2018;13(12):e0208107.
9. Marcus U, Ort J, Grenz M, et al. Risk factors for HIV and STI diagnosis in a community-based HIV/STI testing and counselling site for men having sex with men (MSM) in a large German city in 2011-2012. BMC Infect Dis 2015; 15(14):1–8.
10. Centers for Disease Control and Prevention. STDs and HIV – CDC fact sheet 2017. Available at: https://www.cdc.gov/std/hiv/stdfact-std-hiv-detailed.htm. Accessed January 14, 2020.
11. de Vries HJ. Current challenges in the clinical management of sexually transmitted infections. J Int AIDS Soc 2019;22(S6):e25347.
12. Vasanthamoorthy R, Balachandar J. Prevalence of sexually transmitted infections in HIV seropositive individuals in a rural tertiary care centre in South India. J Evid Based Med Healthc 2018;5(53):3678–81.
13. Mayer KH, Venkatesh KK. Interactions of HIV, other sexually transmitted diseases, and genital tract inflammation facilitating local pathogen transmission and acquisition. Am J Reprod Immunol 2011;65(3):308–16.
14. Cohen MS, Council OD, Chen JS, et al. Sexually transmitted infections and HIV in the era of antiretroviral treatment and prevention: the biologic basis for epidemiologic synergy. J Int AIDS Soc 2019;22(S6):e25355.
15. Mwatelah R, McKinnon LR, Baxter C, et al. Mechanisms of sexually transmitted infection-induced inflammation in women: implications for HIV risk. J Int AIDS Soc 2019;22(S6):e25346.

16. Bamniya J, Singh P, Deora A, et al. A study of prevalence of lower genital tract infections in HIV positive females-a cross sectional study. Int J Reprod Contracept Obstet Gynecol 2017;6(2):645–8.

17. Buckner LR, Amedee AM, Albritton HL, et al. Chlamydia trachomatis infection of endocervical epithelial cells enhances early HIV transmission events. PLoS One 2016;11(1):e0146663.

18. Adachi K, Klausner JD, Bristow CC, et al. Chlamydia and gonorrhea in HIV-infected pregnant women and infant HIV transmission. Sex Transm Dis 2015; 42(10):554–65.

19. Taylor MM, Newman DR, Gonzalez J, et al. HIV status and viral loads among men testing positive for rectal gonorrhoea and chlamydia, Maricopa County, Arizona, USA, 2011-2013. HIV Med 2015;16(4):249–54.

20. Adachi K, Xu J, Yeganeh N, et al. Combined evaluation of sexually transmitted infections in HIV-infected pregnant women and infant HIV transmission. PLoS One 2018;13(1):e0189851.

21. Kidd S, Bowen VB, Torrone EA, et al. Use of national syphilis surveillance data to develop a congenital syphilis prevention cascade and estimate the number of potential congenital syphilis cases averted. Sex Transm Dis 2018;45(9): S23–8.

22. Taylor MM, Newman DR, Schillinger JA, et al. Viral loads among HIV-infected persons diagnosed with primary and secondary syphilis in 4 US cities: New York City, Philadelphia, PA, Washington, DC, and Phoenix, AZ. J Acquir Immune Defic Syndr 2015;70(2):179–85.

23. Looker KJ, Elmes JA, Gottlieb SL, et al. Effect of HSV-2 infection on subsequent HIV acquisition: an updated systematic review and meta-analysis. Lancet Infect Dis 2017;17(12):1303–16.

24. Looker KJ, Margaret AM, Turner KM, et al. Global estimates of prevalent and incident herpes simplex virus type 2 infections in 2012. PLoS One 2015;10(1): e114989.

25. Keller MJ, Huber A, Espinoza L, et al. Impact of herpes simplex virus type 2 and human immunodeficiency virus dual infection on female genital tract mucosal immunity and the vaginal microbiome. J Infect Dis 2019;220(5):852–61.

26. Domercant JW, Louis FJ, Hulland E, et al. Seroprevalence of herpes simplex virus type-2 (HSV-2) among pregnant women who participated in a national HIV surveillance activity in Haiti. BMC Infect Dis 2017;17(1):577.

27. Bradley J, Floyd S, Piwowar-Manning E, et al. Sexually transmitted bedfellows: exquisite association between HIV and herpes simplex virus type 2 in 21 communities in Southern Africa in the HIV prevention trials network 071 (PopART) Study. J Infect Dis 2018;218(3):443–52.

28. Katz DA, Dombrowski JC, Bell TR, et al. HIV incidence among men who have sex with men after diagnosis with sexually transmitted infections. Sex Transm Dis 2016;43(4):249–54.

29. Joseph Davey DL, Nyemba DC, Gomba Y, et al. Prevalence and correlates of sexually transmitted infections in pregnancy in HIV-infected and-uninfected women in Cape Town, South Africa. PLoS One 2019;14(7): e0218349.

30. Champredon D, Bellan SE, Delva W, et al. The effect of sexually transmitted co-infections on HIV viral load amongst individuals on antiretroviral therapy: a systematic review and meta-analysis. BMC Infect Dis 2015;15(1):1–11.

31. de Melo MG, Sprinz E, Gorbach PM, et al. HIV-1 heterosexual transmission and association with sexually transmitted infections in the era of treatment as prevention. Int J Infect Dis 2019;87:128–34.

32. World Health Organization. Report on global sexually transmitted infection surveillance 2018. 2018. Available at: https://www.who.int/reproductivehealth/publications/stis-surveillance-2018/en. Accessed February 8, 2020.

33. Workowski KA, Bolan GA. Sexually transmitted diseases treatment guidelines, 2015. MMWR Recomm Rep 2015;64(3):1–134.

Moving?

Make sure your subscription moves with you!

To notify us of your new address, find your **Clinics Account Number** (located on your mailing label above your name), and contact customer service at:

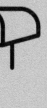

Email: journalscustomerservice-usa@elsevier.com

800-654-2452 (subscribers in the U.S. & Canada)
314-447-8871 (subscribers outside of the U.S. & Canada)

Fax number: 314-447-8029

Elsevier Health Sciences Division
Subscription Customer Service
3251 Riverport Lane
Maryland Heights, MO 63043

*To ensure uninterrupted delivery of your subscription, please notify us at least 4 weeks in advance of move.

ELSEVIER

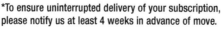